To Do No Harm

Learning to
Care for
the Seriously Ill

Alan C. Mermann

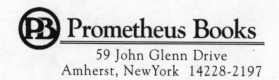
Prometheus Books
59 John Glenn Drive
Amherst, NewYork 14228-2197

Published 1999 by Humanity Books, an imprint of Prometheus Books

03 02 01 00 99   5 4 3 2 1

Library of Congress Cataloging-in-Publication Data

Mermann, Alan C., 1923–
    To do no harm : Learning to care for the seriously ill / Alan C. Mermann.
        p.   cm.
    Includes bibliographical references.
    ISBN 1–57392–666–3 (paper : alk. paper). —ISBN 1–57392–667–1 (cloth : alk. paper)
    1. Critically ill—Care. 2. Terminal care. I. Title.
R726.8.M46   1999
362.1'75—dc21   99–10115
                                                                        CIP

This book is dedicated to my teachers:
physicians at Johns Hopkins,
patients and parents in my practice,
my students at Yale,
our patient-teachers,
and
my four daughters.
All of them taught me the many
and varied aspects of compassion and caring.

Contents

Introduction

It hath been often said, that it is not death,
but dying which is terrible.
　　　　　　　　—Henry Fielding, *Amelia* (1751)

During this past decade, questions about how we die increased dramatically. A topic considered taboo since the Victorian Age is now a subject of open discussion, theological pronouncement, ethical argument, and legislative debate. There are many opinions about choices offered and actions taken. Morality; professional duty and responsibility; costs in money, time, and resources; the harsh realities of suffering, pain, and sorrow—these various factors influence our prejudices, expectations, and decisions about ourselves and those for whom we accept the final responsibility of care and, often, of decisions about living or dying. The reasons for this new and intense interest in end-of-life judgments are important for our consideration, and we find their source in a new and developing medical technology that allows the human body to be kept "alive" with diminished or absent mental functions as we ordinarily think of them. This impressive scientific advance, so essential in emergency situations such as accidents, stroke, and heart attack where recovery is possible, even probable, forces us to rethink old notions of what it means to be a person. Questions are asked now that were unimaginable in the recent past. We are concerned now about what it means to be a person; what are the characteristics of being both an individual and a responsible member of society? We are confronted with dilemmas, with situations where choices must be made, and made by many of us without time for considered deliberation and discussion. As a result of these changes, more and more of us find ourselves thinking through what it means to be a person today. We realize that our decisions about how we die—we and those we care for—will be clear statements about how we understand life, both as persons and as members of a community.

In 1982 I retired from the practice of medicine after twenty-eight years to become the chaplain to the Yale University School of Medicine. I graduated from Yale Divinity School and was ordained a minister in the United Church of Christ in 1979. As one would in a new position, I spent my first months at the medical school listening to students talk about their training: their studies and their experiences with teachers and patients. They said that, in their four years of medical education, they saw a distinct transition between the second and third years. The first two years—called the preclinical years—are focused on the basic biomedical sciences: anatomy, physiology, biochemistry, pathology, pharmacology, and others. The third and fourth years are the clinical years when patient care is taught in hospital rotations in surgery, internal medicine, pediatrics, psychiatry, and obstetrics and gynecology. Students take elective courses and subinternships in fields they are considering as specialties. This is usually the period, also, when the thesis required for graduation is completed.

The transition between the preclinical and the clinical years was described as a disturbing one for many students. As they talked in my office, I learned of the disappointments many students experience in their learning to care for patients. Their primary teachers are the house staff—resident physicians and surgeons—who are often fatigued and stressed by the difficulties of their work, and whose central concern is patient care, not teaching. Attending physicians, usually highly committed to demanding research, the need to acquire funding through grants, and administrative responsibilities, are not readily available to students beginning to learn basic skills of history taking and physical examination. As students observe the practice of medicine and surgery in the hospital, they learn the importance placed on laboratory results, the need to master technical skills such as drawing blood and doing spinal taps, and the importance of case presentations on rounds, all these inferred directly by the staff. Recognizing the importance of these factors in patient care, the students nevertheless felt that other skills—caring for persons who are sick, disabled, despairing, dying, or merely lonely and frightened—should be taught as part of the duties and responsibilities of the good physician.

There are a number of personal characteristics of patients that are important to their care, although often ignored by healthcare personnel. There is a considerable gulf between the education and the training of a subspecialist—a neurosurgeon, for instance—and many of the persons who need that special care. Social-class ethnic factors are important determinants of our behavior, often poorly understood by physicians and surgeons in an academic environment sharply focused on research, technology, and unusual diseases and new treatments. While there are profound changes in the biomedical sciences that reflect in the care provided in medical centers, many doctors still practice more according to their experience than to newly published studies and therapy trials. Experience over time seems to be a strong determinant of both treatment and interaction with patients. Another factor in understanding illness that may be ignored by the doctor is the patient's perception of the disease, its causes and effects, that can be very helpful in planning treatment. Conversations are often stilted, one-directional, and brief, discounting, through ignorance, some of the abiding fears patients live with daily. The popularity of alternative medical treatments suggests that sincere and informed understanding of the interpretations patients have of their diseases must be credited. The more support the physician offers, the more satisfaction and confidence will be elicited from the patient. Neil Kessel, in the Department of Psychiatry at the University of Manchester, writing in the British journal *Lancet* about reassurance, notes,

Reassurance encourages hope and, through the confidence engendered, it enhances the doctor-patient relationship so that partnership can work effectively. It makes patients better able to bear what must be borne, both of illness and of treatment . . . and successful reassurance promotes a patient's wellbeing. . . . The doctor should understand the patient as an individual, appreciate his feelings and his fears and the efforts he is making. The doctor may wish to consider the patient's condition within medical terms of reference—that is, pathological process. The patient's terms of reference embody what he is actually going through and he will not be reassured unless he believes that the doctor is sensitive to, and understands, that.[1]

Some students told me of their distress at the loss of their sense of calling to a caring profession; they felt sharp and uncomfortable changes in the hopes and promises they spoke of when they entered medical school; of anticipating being with and for the sick and the sad. One of the stumbling blocks the students noted was their own difficulty they had in talking about the serious personal issues of their patients. They felt qualified to discuss laboratory results, X-ray studies, and physical findings. But what these findings mean—what the disease means to the patient as person—this was transmitted badly, if at all. How do we talk to anxious others about these things when we are anxious and untrained ourselves? Talking with others about confusing, even ambiguous, findings of examinations, treatments, and outlooks for the future is demanding and difficult. There are social attitudes toward certain diseases—AIDS, cancer, epilepsy—that are negative and hurtful, and carry the stigma of unacceptance. There are poignant, painful, and occasionally hurtful relationships between dying persons and their relatives and friends that may require resolution. Support and suggestions for coping with the stresses of hospitalization, loss, and suffering are needs many of us will have. Training in these areas is commonly minimal.

Another negative factor for medical students in many schools is the expressed need for students to prepare themselves to "survive" medical school. This word is a common one in describing the coming years of education and training. It was a new concept for me, trained as I was in another time and in a different environment. When I arrived at the medical school, entering students received a *Survival Kit,* an attractive information guide on how to get through school with minimal trauma. It also told where the best pizza is to be found, and where the movies and bars are! But Yale was not alone; this is a common practice in medical schools and there are books published and available on how to survive medical school. As I put these assorted observations together, I realized that I was hearing feelings of inadequacy in talking with patients about what was happening to them as persons, as individuals with families and friends, with work and play, with hopes and dreams, with fears and dread. A first task was to delete "survival" from the name of the booklet, leaving it as *The Kit.*

One of the reasons for becoming a doctor is a hope, a seriously thought-through desire to comfort and support others when they are sick and alienated from their personal and social worlds, even from their interior and intimate selves. How can one learn this type of personal and professional involvement and commitment in an environment where science and technology are dominant and very important factors in a profession? I went over to the hospital and talked with some very sick patients and told them what I was hearing in my office. I explained my somewhat vague goal: showing anxious students that we can talk about the personal aspects of disease openly and candidly. The patients understood this immediately, of course, and were pleased to be part of this exercise. After doing this for a few months, it was obvious that the students could—indeed, should—be doing this themselves. The two initial categories were persons with leukemia or metastatic cancer and persons with AIDS. These patients offered a broad spectrum of experience: a grandparent with slowly spreading prostate cancer; a graduate student with leukemia; a professor with AIDS. The students were introduced to concentric circles of families, friends, colleagues, and society. Out of this original experiment developed the Seminar on the Seriously Ill Patient in which the student is the interviewer, the learner; the experiences are the source material for this study.

This book will review the decade of those experiences and that learning. I will also look at interview information that I gathered from physicians and surgeons who do very difficult and trying work, looking for the resources caregivers use for support when the work is challenging and so often depressing in outcome. In this study of ways to learn how to care for seriously ill and dying persons, the goal is the development in all of us of ways of understanding our selves, our work, and our relationships to others and to our world. This understanding will be grounded in a variety of complex and intriguing foundations: philosophy, science, religion, spirituality, psychology, and our social networks. We learn of these foundations by conversation with others farther along on life's journey, by study of classical and contemporary texts, and by contemplation of, and reflection upon, our own experiences and commitments. As we construct our own lives as caregivers, as relational persons, and as social citizens, we are preparing ourselves to face those ultimate questions of life and its values that all of us will meet. The roles we all play as caregivers, as students, and ultimately as patients will be studied from a personal perspective, encouraging a moral, spiritual, and intellectual investigation of the self that will show our clearest definition of who we are to ourselves and to others. The final goal of this study is learning the possibilities and the joys of an examined life that allow us to face its end with equanimity and confidence. The decisions we will make in regard to the varied ways of meeting that end should be informed by thought and conversations well in advance of the final moments. The details of that ending will be confirmed by what we know of ourselves and the foundation we choose to support our life.

Note

1. N. Kessel, "Reassurance," *Lancet*, no. 1 (1979): 1128, 1131.

1

"I Can't Believe I Did That!"

S he walked into my office with a stricken look on her face, dropped into the chair next to my desk, and burst into tears. I learned, during thirty years of medical practice as a pediatrician, to sit and wait for the story soon to be told. She was a third-year student several months into the clinical rotations that are our introduction to the practice of the art and science of medicine. In this third, or clinical, year, students are taught the basics: to interview; take a history and do a physical examination on the patients assigned to them; learn to interpret signs, symptoms, and laboratory findings; and know current treatment possibilities for the diseases they see and study. There are daily conferences, or rounds, where the progress and treatments of the patients are discussed and evaluated by attending physicians, resident physicians (house officers), nurses, social workers, and students. This is a crucial learning site for students; whatever else is said in lecture or read in textbooks, it is on rounds that the medical student learns how medicine is practiced: it is here that the vocabulary and the "ways and the means" of the inner sanctum of the profession are spelled out for the student. This third year is an exciting time of anticipation and of apprehension as the student gets a forward look in time and *sees* the future doctor-to-be. This is as true for psychiatry as it is for surgery, as valid for internal medicine as it is for obstetrics and gynecology. Regardless of profession, we learn the tricks of the trade by observing those senior to us in experience and knowledge.

This student came to see me because we had talked in the past about why she wanted to become a doctor. She, along with many of her peers, was drawn to medicine as a career because it is a profession that, in its higher moments, is dedicated to caring for others who are sick, be it in body or mind. She had the required intellect, and also the interest and education in the sciences and the humanities. Medicine offered both the opportunity to care for the sick and the sufferers, and the intellectual challenges of a profession with a strong foundation in new sciences. During her first two preclinical years of study in the biological sciences we talked about the goals of medicine, the delights and stresses of patient-physician interactions, and the deep personal satisfactions possible for a trained and competent physician. We also talked about the profoundly difficult personal issues in medicine. How can one continue to care for persons who do not care for themselves? How do we maintain a professional and attentive attitude toward drug users, prostitutes, drunks, heavy smokers, and food addicts? What is the personal, internal foundation that we need to be physicians for those who use and abuse the system, seem to have no moral base in their lives, and dislike, even despise, us?

And now, here she was, crying in my office. Her first words were, "I can't believe I did that!" What she had done was refer to a patient with the epithet "dirtball." After all her conversations about the need to respect each patient as a fellow human being on the journey of life, the requirement that we set aside the negative personal and behavioral aspects of our patients and attend to the medical needs presented to us, and her insistence on our basic commitment to care for all without prejudice, she had learned—and used—the language of disrespect for another person. Her shame and her concern for her behavior were quite evident and alarmed her. We talked about her dismay, and I assured her, as best I could, that these humbling experiences can help us grow and mature when we recognize what we have done, and the context within which it took place. She had learned quite unconsciously from her teachers—attending and resident physicians—to use degrading language and acronyms to label and denigrate others. Her education was insidious and, probably, unintentional, but real nevertheless. It would take time, thought, and an appreciation of this new and painfully acquired self-knowledge to undo the damage she had experienced. This new knowledge could alert her to future danger signals in her interactions with teachers and patients.

Medical Students

At this beginning of our study of how we learn to care for the seriously ill, it will be helpful to have some information about medical students, those who are on their way to becoming doctors. Who does become a doctor? Do they have defining characteristics; are they different from other graduate students? We need a baseline from which to understand and appreciate the impressive personal qualities, the intelligence, the commitments, and the skills that these young people bring to the profession. We also need to understand some of the personality characteristics of medical students that influence, and actually determine, the type of physician we are training. There is no generic medical student; as with all of us, each is an individual with idiosyncrasies, personality traits, anxieties, aspirations, and inheritances of mind and body that determine our differences, one from the other. Studies have been done of university students in the various graduate schools that document some differences in the ways that medical and other graduate students look at ethical and moral questions. These studies also consider the influences of medical education and clinical training upon moral development. These studies are not definitive of any individual, but they do provide a starting point for looking at personality traits of the doctors who will care for us when we are sick.

As we look at how we are trained to care for the sick, I will present a brief, and certainly incomplete, overview—a vignette, perhaps—of some of the hallmarks of young women and men studying

to become doctors. This can assist us in understanding some of the
attitudes of students and doctors, the startling changes that occurred
in the young woman noted above, and reasons for my concerns about
how we learn to care for seriously ill persons. Medical education and
training are probably the strongest influences that alter the personality of a graduate student and bring that person to professional
maturity. There are multiple factors involved—many positive and
some destructive—that influence, and finally control, the construct of
the physician. I present some of these studies as background information to allay any questions that casual observation or personal bias
determine my work.

In 1967 Kenneth Keniston, a psychologist in the Department of
Psychiatry at the Yale University School of Medicine, published an
article, "The Medical Student." In this study, one that I believe
remains seminal for us, he discusses a variety of distinguishing traits
of students that give us a framework for understanding the person
beginning the transformation into a doctor. Keniston notes three
psychological themes of students that draw them to medicine as a
profession:

> (1) [M]edical students are frequently individuals with a long-
> standing need for, enjoyment of, capacity to tolerate being in a
> caring, providing, dispensing, nurturing relationship to other
> people. . . . (2) It is not uncommon for medical students to have
> chosen medicine after a death of a family member or close friend,
> sometimes with the quite conscious desire to learn how to fight
> wasteful death. . . . (3) [I]ntimate personal contact with physical or
> psychological suffering, whether in themselves or in others, seems
> to have disposed other students toward a vocation in which their
> lives will be partly devoted to combatting suffering.[1]

These concerns are certainly not limited to medical students, but
they play strong roles in their understanding of their future careers as
doctors. They are instrumental in drawing women and men to medicine as a career. The number of applicants to medical schools is high,
and the qualifications of these undergraduates are impressive, indeed.

As a member of the admissions committee of the Yale School of Medicine, I can attest to the importance of the themes noted above. Most applicants are talented in several fields, have done volunteer service, participated in research projects, and speak to a strong commitment to the possibilities that medicine holds for living a life of good works and sincere service. The hopes they hold to help patients is, interestingly, limited more to personalized care than it is to the community in general. A study of students at Oregon Health Sciences University Medical School published in 1993 confirms this impression, with students hoping to provide personal care and develop positive relationships with patients. This finding is parallel to their hopes for a realized self-fulfillment as physicians, and personal challenges and variety in that work. Not unexpectedly, contact with the suffering of a friend or family member would dispose us toward a career that could work toward alleviating that suffering. The authors write, "Of note, the most common hope of first-year medical students is to help others. Also of interest is that responses relating to hopes about making an 'impact on the local community' or 'impact on general society' were relatively infrequent."[2]

Keniston finds that medical students are distinguished by the methods they employ to adapt to life events. Anxiety, a feeling common in human experiences, is dealt with by efforts to counter and master the anxiety by overcoming its sources. They tend to react to stress by efforts to change the environment, rather than altering their responses to it. This seems to be a less effective method of coping with the inevitable stresses of caring for sick persons, particularly when there are so many unknowns in diagnosis and treatment, and unanswerable questions about prognosis. The management of ambiguity and uncertainty in medical practice, tied as they are to the vagaries of human existence, is a major concern. The constant changes in technology and biomedical sciences force upon us the need for ongoing study and reassessment of our skills. In a study measuring the coping skills of senior and first-year students at three medical schools published in the journal *Medical Education* in 1994, the authors note that the emphasis on biophysical models of disease has encouraged reliance upon science and decreased the ability to tolerate uncertainty.

> Outcomes in clinical medicine cannot be reduced to a simple suc-
> cess or failure alternative. Teachers have a responsibility to teach
> their students that in treating patients, "success" has many defini-
> tions. If medical students' abilities to manage ambiguity are to be
> improved, medical educators need to examine how they are
> moulding students' success expectancy. . . .[3]

Medical education cannot address only the biological aspects of
illness. The interior, exquisitely individualistic, and completely
unique aspects of being a person make medical care a profound challenge. We all have habits, beliefs, convictions, and attitudes that,
however eccentric, are ours and must be taken into account as part of
any treatment plan. And it is grasping the significance of this partic-
ularity that must be understood as a part of the treatment of the
whole person. A premier American physician at the turn of the century who addressed some of these challenges and enigmas of medicine was William Osler. In a time when quackery was widespread and
medical education generally poor, definitive therapies were rare.
Surgery, when anesthesia and antisepsis were finally acceptable,
advanced rapidly. Medical treatments were marginally valuable, often
harmful. As a result, well-trained physicians of the time honed their
diagnostic skills and learned to *care* for sick persons, knowing that
little could be done to *cure*. A personality characteristic that Osler
encouraged as a way of managing the self in caring for others was
equanimity. In his famous valedictory address, "Aequanimitas," to
students graduating from the University of Pennsylvania in 1889 he
comments on our patients, our fellow travelers,

> full of fads and eccentricities, of whims and fancies; but the more
> closely we study their little foibles of one sort and another in the
> inner life which we see, the more surely is the conviction borne in
> upon us of the likeness of their weaknesses to our own. . . . A dis-
> tressing feature in the life which you are about to enter . . . is the
> uncertainty which pertains not alone to our science and art, but to
> the very hopes and fears which make us men.[4]

Osler encouraged his students and residents to identify themselves with those in their care. The very richness of life possible to the physician lies hidden like a treasure in our identification with patients, those companions on our common journey whom we are called to attend.

There are stresses in the practice of medicine that can be nearly overwhelming, and coping skills must be taught early so that the developing student can remain well and contribute to the general health. Failure to do so can have damaging effects on the prospective doctor. In a study of third-year students at the University of Mississippi Medical Center published in 1994 in *Academic Medicine*, coping methods that engage the student—learning, expression of emotion, problem solving, and seeking support—were found to be helpful and effective in preventing depression. Contrary methods that cause disengagement—withdrawal, wishful thinking, and avoidance of issues—are detrimental to the student.[5] Obviously, teaching students the ways and means of positive engagement with problems—clinical or personal—will help in the development of caring physicians. One of the concerns is that these interior and personal skills are often not taught to students because they are either not important or not accessible to the faculty.

For persons for whom acceptance by a medical school is highly determined by grade-point averages and scores on national examinations, an intellectual response to troubling feelings seems an expected course to follow. Unfortunately, this approach can be harmful to the development of empathy and compassionate feelings toward suffering persons. For some students, this expressed need for, and enjoyment of, caring and nurturant relationships and a wish to fight wasteful death are diminished by negative attitudes toward others. As an example, a study of medical students in five California schools published in 1995 shows that entering students already possess less favorable attitudes toward older persons. The study finds difficulty in predicting and identifying these attitudes in prospective applicants, although males and Asian students were more likely to be prejudiced against older persons. The authors write, "the focus of efforts to generate physicians with good attitudes must rely on curricular efforts during medical school and residency training."[6] This finding runs counter to what we would expect: if experience with disease and death in family or close friends draws one to a career in medicine, we would expect that relationships with parents and grandparents should draw us toward, rather than turn us away from, older persons. Of course, the autobiographical sketch and the experiences recorded in the personal essay in an application to medical school are not necessarily completely accurate.

The disengagement of many students from their feelings is a major source of concern for teaching compassionate care for seriously ill persons, particularly when death is a distinct and recognized probability. Self-study is not a characteristic of students highly trained in the sciences; their thoughts are directed outward toward "things" as objects of study. Keniston finds that

> medical students are notable for the speed and zeal with which they attempt to devise practical, well-organized plans for changing things; they seem to be less inclined to examine their own motives, feelings, and fantasies, much less to advocate self-reform before reform of the world. Finally, and perhaps most impressive, medical students, like many other students with developed scientific ability, generally possess a considerable capacity to translate feelings into ideas, to manipulate these ideas, and at times to forget the feelings that originally underlay them.[7]

The result, unfortunate for both student and future patients, is dismissal of feelings that are bothersome. One of the goals in medical education must be the recognition that our personal responses to our world and to our work must be addressed as such, not converted into a theoretical problem for the intellect. Medical students learn an astounding amount of factual material, techniques, and scientific reasoning. They also learn adaptive skills that are not conducive to sympathetic and personal attitudes toward patients, particularly if the patient is a social outcast, a person of questionable moral status, or has a lifestyle believed to be the cause of the medical problem presented. Use of drugs, alcoholism, criminal behavior, and smoking are behavioral patterns that can result in personal rejection by students and staff. Why work hard and long for patients who return again and again because of their negative lifestyles and disdain for the system?

Associated with the psychological models and techniques of coping noted above, there can be damping of personal responses to friends, social concerns, and to the power of sexuality and intimacy necessary for a realized personal social life with some degree of fullness. The very skills of dissociation from feelings learned in cadaver dissection, examination of breast and rectum, and other extremely personal encounters can repress the feelings that we should normally expect to have, be they revulsion, curiosity, or sympathy. Students often note with dismay this retreat from feelings, as do their friends in other graduate academic fields. The results of this neutralizing process can be damaging to future family development and social commitments to changes in our environments, personal, social, and ecological. Sad to say, clinical depression and marital problems are well known among physicians in training.

The educational process in medical school has a deciding effect upon moral development. In a small study of students using the Kohlberg Moral Judgment Interview, a 1993 report published in *Medical Education* documents a definite tendency for students to move toward a median level of moral reasoning; those testing high and those testing low both move toward the middle over the four years. "The trends in the data demonstrate that the range of moral judgement scores of the students decrease after 4 years of medical education, indicating a strong socializing factor. . . ." The results—students in higher levels of reasoning dropping, and those in lower levels rising—"indicate a movement toward homogeneity in moral thinking that may be due to the medical education experience."[8] Of interest also is that other students of the same age and level of education in the United States do not show the same narrowing move toward the middle. It seems obvious that education and exposure to the models available in medical school have defining effects upon the level of moral reasoning graduating doctors will have attained. In this study there were no outstanding differences related to gender, although changes that occurred, particularly regression, seemed more prominent in women.

A central tenet of my belief and a conviction based upon my experiences as physician and as an instructor is that we learn our ethics and our moral standards by observing our mentors, not by classroom lecture. Ethical dilemmas—those moments of decision when there is no clearcut right or wrong—presented in medical practice offer opportunities for teaching by example. Unfortunately, the old saw "Do as I say, not as I do" is a common occurrence. In a study of ethical erosion in third-year students in six Pennsylvania medical schools published in 1994 in *Academic Medicine*, the authors comment,

> The present survey suggests that many students confront dilemmas that are shaped by their subordinate role within the hierarchical medical team. While wrestling with such predicaments may encourage some students to mature into thoughtful and ethical physicians, our analysis indicates that, for at least a sizable minority, exposures to student-level dilemmas coincide with deterioration of the students' ethical self-identities.[9]

A most distressing coincidental finding was that some students "reported that their principles had been eroded but were not displeased with their ethical development, as though they have accepted that becoming a doctor requires a transformation of character."[10]

Major changes in medical and surgical practice and in the teaching of students and staff followed the end of World War II. Amazing technological advances, the development of antibiotics, federal support for research, and an enthusiasm for the future were exciting. The role of the physician shifted from personal care for the sick to using the new diagnostic and therapeutic tools available. One of the responses to the sensed alienation of doctors from the personal needs of their patients was the introduction of courses in the humanities and biomedical ethics in medical schools. A wide variety of topics are addressed in attempts to improve medical care and the personal satisfaction to be known in practicing medicine. Success has been limited. In discussing this addition to the medical curriculum, a report from the University of Virginia published in *Academic Medicine* in 1994 concludes "that formal course work in medical ethics has a limited influence on medical students."[11] The basic education in the ethical and moral practice of medicine, that is, the proper care of seriously ill patients, is the responsibility of those who teach, the surgeons and physicians taking care—in the literal sense of that word—of patients. The attitudes and beliefs of the faculty will determine the attributes of the future physicians toward patients. In a commentary published in *Theoretical Medicine* in 1995, Brody, Squier, and Foglio conclude their discussion on moral growth in medical students with this observation:

> The task of moral growth and development require that our current attitudes and behaviors be situated within the larger framework of our lives. . . . But we cannot meaningfully discuss issues of virtue, integrity, and character without talking about what it means to live a complete life, to aspire to live one's life in accord with a core set of values, and to strive *to behave in such a way that one's behavior embodies those core value commitments.*[12] (Italics mine)

In other words, compassionate care sensitive to the total needs of the patient, honest and kind attention to the humanity of those in our care, and integrity in the teaching of medicine can only be taught successfully by example. Clinical and technical skills are critical in caring for others; how we "attend" our patients will determine not only their care, but our satisfaction and contentment with our choice of work. But the clinician is not the sole teacher of the student. The patient is an essential source for learning how to be a good doctor. This observation, which seems simplistic at first, will be developed in detail in this study.

The Clinical Years

Joining the "team" taking care of patients is a heady experience. Not only does the student use the techniques of taking a history and examining a patient, discuss possible diagnoses, and suggest treatments, one becomes a functional member of the team that is caring for sick persons. The student also learns that performance in the hospital is detailed in the evaluations sent to the office of the dean for student affairs. These evaluations are of critical importance for the letters sent out to hospitals to which fourth-year students will apply for residency training. The result is that medical students pay attention to the wishes, practices, orders, and suggestions of the attending and resident physicians, most of which are relevant to medical care, not personal issues around illness. In this environment, intelligent and alert students pay attention.

The fatigue of an overworked house staff, the importance of laboratory results, attending physicians who are supported by grants and income generated by outpatient faculty practice and not by ward attending: these facts can seriously limit the opportunities for students to observe the defining characteristics of the surgeon or physician they thought they were coming to medical school to become. Students learn that many members of the staff have little interest in the personal concerns of their patients. Questions about the future, about anxiety and fear, about the impact of serious disease upon all the aspects of a life—these often have a very low priority for doctors and are turned over to social workers and other staff. By observing the medical staff students learn how they are to behave, what the criteria are for success, and the core values of physicians.

The patient is the source of our learning because there is a unique character to each one. Language and beliefs—all parts of our culture—not only speak to how we know we are sick, but also why we are sick. There are patterns to our understanding of events that differ; if the caregiver is disinterested or unaware, crucial opportunities for serving the sick can be lost. We need to elicit the concepts patients have of their disease—causes, alternative explanations for symptoms, other options for treatment—so that patients will understand that we do not regard them as irrational, unsophisticated, or primitive.

One of the distressing observations documented by medical sociologists is the inverse relation between the severity of the illness of a patient and the amount of time the physician spends with that patient. As patients get sicker and medical skills become less important than caring skills, the visits to the room of the patient become remarkably shortened. As patients are dying, care and support become nursing responsibilities, not defining professional functions of the physician. This sends a very clear message to the student about the role of the doctor in caring for the sick.

Who Can Teach Us?

In listening to third-year students discuss their surprise and dismay at the behavior of some of the doctors toward their patients, and their own difficulties in talking with very sick persons, I realized that they needed to be shown that it is possible to communicate in significant personal depth with patients. In fact, hearing the story of another's life is a gift to be valued and treasured. As noted previously, I brought students with me to observe my conversation with a patient hospital-ized with a disease with a very poor prognosis. After introductions, the patient and I begin to talk about the impact of serious disease upon life.

A. B. is seventy years old and has had leukemia for two years. He is admitted with a high fever, and has been told that his bone marrow has not returned to a condition where he can have further chemotherapy at this time. It seems to him, he says, that his time is running out. His wife is there, and they note, with sad smiles, that their conversations have, subtly, but clearly, shifted into the past tense. Where, before, they spoke of plans to see grandchildren, take a short vacation trip, or continue their walking tour of the city, now they talk about their relationship over the years. As the students and I listen, we hear an account of two lives lived, of the sources of strength and courage used to persist in the losing battle against inexorable loss. We learn the characteristics of the good physi-cian, the significance of the touch of a hand, the pause to comment on the "get-well card" from a faraway son. We need ask very few questions; the couple are pleased to teach us of their experiences with this implacable horror that they face with fortitude and a bit of humor. They tell us they are pleased to be part of our learning, and they wish us well.

After a few months of these interviews, I set up a course for first-year students, the Seminar on the Seriously Ill Patient, in which I was the facilitator, not the interviewer. The students took over that task and their education began.

Notes

1. K. Keniston, "The Medical Student," *Yale Journal of Biology and Medicine* 19 (June 1967): 349.

2. S. A. Fields and W. L. Toffler, "Hopes and Concerns of a First-Year Medical School Class," *Medical Education* 27 (1993): 127.

3. J. M. Merrill, Z. Camacho, L. F. Laux, R. Lorimer, J. I. Thornby, and C. Vallbona, "Uncertainties and Ambiguities: Measuring How Medical Students Cope," *Medical Education* 28 (1994): 321.

4. W. Osler, "Aequanimitas," in *Aequanimitas with Other Addresses to Medical Students, Nurses and Practitioners of Medicine* (Philadelphia: P. Blakiston's Son & Co., 1925), 6–7.

5. T. H. Mosley Jr., S. G. Perrin, S. N. Neral, P. M. Dubbert, C. A. Grothues, and B. M. Pinto, "Stress, Coping, and Well-being Among Third-year Medical Students," *Academic Medicine* 69, no. 9 (1994): 765–67.

6. D. B. Reuben, J. T. Fullerton, J. M. Tschann, and M. Croughan-Minihane, "Attitudes of Beginning Medical Students Toward Older Persons: A Five-Campus Study," *JAGS* 43 (1995):1435.

7. Keniston, "The Medical Student," 349.

8. D. J. Self, D. E. Schrader, D. C. Baldwin Jr., and F. D. Wolinsky, "The Moral Development of Medical Students: A Pilot Study of the Possible Influence of Medical Education," *Medical Education* 27 (1993): 32.

9. C. Feudtner, D. A. Christakis, and N. A. Christakis, "Do Clinical Clerks Suffer Ethical Erosion? Students' Perceptions of Their Ethical Environment and Personal Development," *Academic Medicine* 69, no. 8 (1994): 677–78.

10. Ibid.

11. A. F. Shorr, R. P. Hayes, and J. F. Finnerty, "The Effect of a Class in Medical Ethics on First-year Medical Students," *Academic Medicine* 69 no. 12 (1994): 999–1000.

12. H. Brody, H. A. Squier, and J. P. Foglio, "Commentary: Moral Growth in Medical Students," *Theoretical Medicine* 16 (1995): 287.

2

"I Mostly Keep It to Myself"

My wife clues in very quickly to how I'm feeling. If I've had a bad day, she knows it and tells me, "Don't take it out on me—leave it somewhere else." So, I mostly keep it to myself.

The experience of this doctor is disturbing. There is a certain poignancy in imagining the interior life of a doctor unable to speak of the loneliness and the frustrations of a day spent in the care of the sick, but it is not an unusual scenario. It does open for us a discussion of the inner being of many physicians who care for seriously ill patients. In our study of how we can learn to be caring and compassionate doctors alert to the multiple, complex, and often conflicting needs of sick persons, the physician is a key player, a major actor in the drama of the patient-physician relationship. In this chapter I will look at some of the personal and interior aspects of the lives of physicians who care for the seriously ill. Some of these are tied closely to personality traits and educational experiences discussed previously.

Medical students become doctors. The many years of formal education and training finally come to an end, and physicians and surgeons proceed to practice, to teach, and to do research. From the

clinical years of medical school on there have been professional interactions with patients who are seriously ill, many of whom died. For
many doctors, their training lacked a systematic and comprehensive
program for teaching the care of the dying patient; their training also
lacked insightful and sensitive teaching about the ways by which the
physician can understand the personal and the private responses that
both patients and their caregivers make to death. Only in the last few
years have medical schools begun to teach the fundamentals of palliative care. Intellectually, we all know that we shall die. We have
known this since early childhood when the family cat died, or we saw
the dead squirrel on the street killed by a car. Although often sup-
pressed in conversation, we do learn about death. As we shall see, dissection of the cadaver in the first months of medical school provides
final and irrefutable evidence.

Contrary to the everyday experiences of many doctors in practice—private or HMO-related—the physicians and surgeons I will
discuss care for the seriously ill, the dying, and the frequent and
trying crises in medicine every day. While it may seem that they are a
selected and, therefore, an atypical group, I would affirm, rather, that
they are classical examples of the varied ways by which we cope with
those interior, secret, and often conflicting emotional problems
inherent in being a physician. By the very nature of the intensity of
their work they provide a focused picture of the coping techniques—
for good or for ill—that doctors use to deal with the stresses of the
profession. These doctors offer us an inside look at the measures
physicians and surgeons use to help them survive the strains of caring
for us when we are very sick. As might be anticipated, these are the
coping techniques many of us use to resolve the inner struggles of
our daily lives; they are just more sharply outlined when caring for the
very ill.

Much of the work of doctors is characterized by ambiguity and
uncertainty. It is an unhappy fact that we recall our failures far more
easily and clearly than we do our successes; in medicine it is certainly
true. The personal stakes are high when one is diagnosing and
treating serious disease. Errors in judgment and in management can
be costly, sometimes disastrous. Responsibilities rest heavily on doc-

tors since an accurate diagnosis and proper treatment may not be all that obvious, even to the best-trained eye. Ambiguity and veiled signs, symptoms and findings are common, deepening the internalized sense of obligation felt by the physician. There is a pervasive sense of vulnerability in the practice of medicine, that feeling that one is rarely sure of all the details of diagnosis, treatment, and looking to the future. Associated with this, and feeding into it, are the devastations one knows when patients do not do well, when disease takes its final toll. These are known to many of us in our roles as parent, child, or member of a community. Even though there is every reason why treatment was unsuccessful, there is a weariness, a sense of failure, when there is irretrievable loss.

I raise this issue of internalization of feelings and its related problem of the difficulties of the doctor in speaking of the impact of medical practice upon the person because they are central to understanding how we can learn to care better for those who are seriously ill. Certainly, the inner life of the physician determines, in large part, the character of that doctor and the responses made to the needs of the sick. The doctor quoted at the beginning of this chapter carries the added burden of living with feelings and emotions that cannot be analyzed, discussed, and, perhaps, laid aside, at least for the moment. To get some perspective on the person of the doctor, I shall examine several factors: (1) educational determinants of the doctor and their impact on that person; (2) training and experience with patients as influences on development of the "self" of the doctor; (3) relations with others, professional and intimate, that determine the developing physician; and (4) culture and religion that influence the self of the doctor.

Education

As first-year medical students will attest, the experience of dissecting a cadaver is work that creates a clear dividing line between them and other graduate students, a line that persists throughout the life of the doctor. When one looks at the education and the training of the doctor, the severity of the stresses of caring for others who are very sick, and the persistent knowledge that one cannot know everything, we understand why doctors feel they are different from other professionals. And it begins in the anatomy laboratory. Taking a scalpel in hand and opening up the chest to expose lungs and heart, or the abdomen to examine and learn the anatomic structure of our bodies by actually seeing and holding its parts—this begins a unique process of separation from so many other persons. Some find the mere thought of this experience repulsive; others are fascinated by the idea, but are glad that others, not they, are doing it. Anatomy dissection is symbolic of the distinct differences that physicians know between their work and the day-to-day experiences of others. Physicians participate in a reality and have a knowledge quite foreign to most other persons, and the anatomy laboratory is the place where this separation begins. As there is no way to prepare oneself for the experience of dissection of another person's body, so there is also no substitute for it. Of course, the details of human anatomy can be memorized from textbooks and computer graphics presentations; it is, however, the contact—both visual and tactile—with an actual human body begun in that first year in medical school that initiates the separation of the medical student from the rest of the human community. It is a variant of the ritual of baptism, a recognizable sign of entrance into the profession. Just as anatomy dissection is a sign of acceptance into a community, it is also a clear sign of the distance separating the physician from the rest of society. The experience is distinctive, and requires a faculty that leads students through orientation and acculturation to ease in their new world.

We are defined by what we do and how we do it. Whether the calling and dedication are to being a parent or a neurosurgeon, a used-car salesman or a priest, our work defines us to ourselves and to the world. In interviewing applicants to medical school, one of the questions discussed in depth is, "Why do you want to be a doctor?" The answers are obviously important and they help in finding students who have commitments to helping others, confidence in biomedical sciences to make our lives better, and a demonstrated willingness to work hard to learn the scientific basis of medical care and the skills needed to practice that care with confidence. The very content of medical education with its voluminous database of factual information in biomedical sciences places severe demands on the learning capabilities of students and of doctors who must continue to be fully informed throughout professional life. Medical training, with its sharp attention to the uncertainties and complications of diagnosis and treatment, teaches awareness of the obvious: doctors care far more than they cure.

Training and the Self

This need to know the current state of the art and the science of medicine can—and perhaps should—become a compulsion for physicians since their professional competence will rest upon their knowledge as well as their experience. Physicians often speak of a strong and persistent striving to be able to *think,* to be proficient at reasoning in times of difficulty and confusion. For many, this can be compulsive; they must know what they are doing in the particular circumstances in which they find themselves. In a sense, this is an inevitable outgrowth of acceptance of responsibility to patients to provide the best care possible in a certain time and place, to do what is needed. For some this can come close to a drive to perfection, to mastery of the profession as the way to prevent catastrophe and error. There seem to be no shortcuts to this mastery; what we might call total immersion is required. A stated goal of many physicians and surgeons is that they not be surprised by unexpected events and findings, that their training and education prepare them for the exigencies of practice, operating room, emergency department, and psychiatric interview. This need for assurance that one has a sense of mastery, an inner confidence that the years of ongoing education and training have been successful in producing a highly competent doctor, can result in a sharp focus on the self. The acceptance of responsibility for one's actions is never more strongly assumed than it is by physicians. The whole course of training has led to that conclusion, reinforcing the strong and acknowledged need for the sense of mastery common to

the highly competent in any field. This can become a drain on the life
and the work of the doctor when too much—even unnecessary—
responsibility is assumed.

It is important to understand the power of this need for professional knowledge and skill that stretches human capabilities to their
limits. One of the terrors in the practice of medicine is that there will
be a decision, an action, a commitment that will be made in error
because the doctor did not know the correct response to be made to
the situation. The risk of error is an integral part of the thought and
the reasoning of the doctor. There is no way by which we can always
know what to do; the assurance we need is that we knew all that
could be known, and the consequences of our actions and decisions
were the results of chance and could not be known beforehand. This
haunting anxiety is a major source of the reasons for continuing medical education, recertification at intervals in specialties, and close association of many physicians with medical schools and their faculties
and laboratories. Another form of expression of concern for doing as
well as possible by continued study is a common hobby of physicians,
study of the history of medicine. For many, it falls into a search for
models of the good doctor in the past—not in terms of specific scientific knowledge that changes with the seasons, but more in the
search for models of the good physician. The history of Western medicine has a scattering of doctors who represent the epitome of caring,
investigating, and openness to the vagaries of change in the worlds of
both patient care and science. They also represent personal models
that clarify the primary responsibility of the doctor to the patient.

One of the personal by-products of this drive toward that sense
of confidence and mastery is isolation from understanding the power
of what I shall call "feelings," those interior sensations and revelations, those "highs and lows" of emotion that move us unexpectedly
and powerfully at the most unexpected times. A common consequence of contemporary medical training is the separation, the distancing, if you will, of emotion from the work at hand. This would
be as true in the office of the psychoanalyst as in the pediatric car-
diothoracic surgery suite. This shutdown of emotion, or at least the
dampening of its effects on professional functioning, is crucial for

doing the work at hand properly and appropriately. But it has the unfortunate secondary effect of providing a way of dealing with emotions and "feelings" in the nonprofessional scenarios of living in our worlds, and dealing with them in diminished and minimalist ways.

The feelings of vulnerability and insecurity that physicians and surgeons know can encourage suppression of those feelings by intellectualizing the environmental scene in which these feelings occur. There is no need to talk about how we feel since we "know" what happened and our role in the event. How we feel about it becomes a discussion of the event, not our inner sense of failure, ineptness, or sadness. This story line produces a person tough on the self, often unaware of the reasons for vague feelings of anger, anxiety, and ennui; unaware, also, of the needs we all have for closure on difficult times in our lives, for confession to self and to others of our inadequacies and longings, for confronting the hazardous road of life that we walk.

Relationships with Others

There are two "others" that I shall consider in looking at the relationships doctors have with other persons: other physicians as colleagues, and intimate members of family and friends. Although I have spent many years as a physician talking with my peers, most of my insights into the ways we relate to others noted in this chapter come from in-depth interviews with other physicians done over the past decade. As the chaplain in a medical school I am interested in ways that future physicians can learn to care for patients in sensitive and rewarding ways, and in resources that physicians can use to enrich their lives both professionally and personally. The physicians and surgeons I interviewed over the years have presented two opposing—even contradictory—views of their ideas of caring for their own needs. They speak of the need to care for oneself so that one can function fully and rewardingly in the profession. Events, accidents, relationships, even joys and pleasures often require closure: we need to know how to incorporate them into ourselves so that we can move on to the next stage of life and work. They speak also, almost in the same breath, of the need to be tough on the self, to demand—as noted above—the very best of themselves in their work. One doctor suggested that the training she had received was similar to the drivenness of the marathon runner preparing to run the race with full commitment of all her personal resources to the goal of completing the race, if not winning it.

In my experience, physicians often speak with colleagues about their work, even when it does not go well. One intensive-care physician said, "I tell everyone about errors that are made. We must all learn from our mistakes. There is nothing to be gained by hiding information from others." Surgeons critically evaluate their work in weekly conferences that study cases that were unexpectedly difficult, or went badly, looking for ways to prevent errors or complications in the future. These Morbidity and Mortality Conferences can be a serious source of anxiety for the doctors, but are considered essential for learning, from the recent past, how to prepare for the vexing and problematic questions not yet asked, and certainly not answered. These conferences are representative of the intense need physicians and surgeons have to continue to learn, particularly from cases where all did not go well. They represent, also, a confidence in professional relationships that allows and demands open discussion of difficult and trying experiences. The role of the trust of colleagues is central to continuing to do the difficult work that doctors are called to do. This trust is, paradoxically, a source of personal difficulty for the doctor. When things go badly for us, either at work or with our relations with others, we have inner feelings that we recognize as anger, fear, shame, sadness, disgust, and weariness. Many of us have difficulty talking easily about these interior feelings; we can be embarrassed by them, ashamed of our weakness in having them, and a host of other responses.

For many doctors, talking with other doctors about the case that did not go well is one way of dealing with the situation. One is reassured that the work was done as well as possible, considering the unexpected complications, that no one else could have done better, or whatever form the reassurances take. But those inner feelings, those expressions of our emotions, do not get spoken and discussed and resolved. They just sit there. As one physician said, "I keep my feelings inside myself; I just wait for them to go away." As we know, they usually do not go away quickly; instead they pollute our relations with others, often those closest to us. This difficulty in speaking of personal feelings, thinking they have been handled by discussion of the medical case with peers, leaves many doctors with a sense of vulnerability, an uneasy recognition of incompleteness, an absence of closure on important events. One of the key issues in this study is the search for ways by which physicians can learn to know and own their feelings; the role of patients as teachers of these skills will be discussed later.

One of the wrenching paradoxes in medicine is living in intimacy with suffering, pain, and death—the human experiences doctors are trained to confront—and knowing that so often little can be done to help. The plight of others with serious, life-threatening diseases can cause us to harden ourselves to our patients. Those same conditions can, however, also provide the locus for a deepened sense of human worth and dignity, a willingness to give of the self to others, and a profound acknowledgment of the gratitude we have for our lives. A pediatric surgeon said that there is a most sobering moment when, as an operation is about to begin, there is the realization that this patient is somebody's child, a boy or girl like one's own, whose very life is in your hands. Not only is the reality of that child placed before us; it could, in other circumstances, be our own child. As the surgeon said, "We have so much, and we do not appreciate it until we truly understand what we are doing." In this way a physician grasps the reality of the calling to be a doctor, understands the blessings of the work, and knows the emotion of gratitude and grace.

Another aspect of medical practice, a function of the profession that is demanding of time, emotion, and thought, is interpreting and understanding the importance of the intimate knowledge doctors have of their patients. Not only the intimacy of the physical examination and current state of health are known. Many physicians are privy to the elemental—occasionally secret—personal, behavioral, and psychological contents of the lives of their patients. This knowledge is held in confidence, moral judgments are set aside, and the expertise of the physician is applied to assist a return to health in all its categories. While this experience may seem like a pleasant one for a voyeur, it is a substantial burden for the doctor to carry. Much of what patients relate of their lives is tragic and sad, revealing the plight of others that cannot be relieved, only heard out and consoled. Again here, as we shall develop later, teaching the lessons of sickness by the patient can be of inestimable value in completing the training of the good doctor.

As noted in the quotation at the opening of this chapter, communication with a spouse about inner feelings can be difficult. The emotional loneliness known to many in the practice of medicine makes any intimate revelations about the self frustrating, often unsuccessful. Medical care of patients with widespread cancer, surgical treatment of heart defects of newborn infants, or efforts to bolster failing hearts and lungs are often futile and end in death. How can one who does this work go home every night and relate the stories of the day to a spouse? As we noted above, the conversations with colleagues dealt with the medical parts of the case; what does the doctor do now with the feelings that swirl through the mind after the event? This problem is common in the interviews I have done over the years: the doctor suppresses the emotions that are present, misunderstanding their import for knowing the self as a person. The lack of clarity about the nature of feelings confuses the situation, making it difficult to speak to what is going on inside. Some spouses are more willing to listen than the doctor is to talk. There is also—common to our culture—usually more willingness and capability of women to talk than men. Also evident in many persons is the inference that when something has not gone well at work, it is the fault of the worker, and we have difficulty entering that arena of talk. Many persons hold back their thoughts, say little about the very things that are bothering them so, and hope that it will all go away. It is this aspect of the life of the doctor that must be addressed far more diligently in the future of medical training. There is a richness in exploring the function of our feelings—good and bad—that leads to a fuller life.

Cultural and Religious Influences

A major concern of mine during this past decade of learning and teaching about ways to improve the relationships between doctors and patients who are very sick is the role that religion and culture play in the professional life of the doctor. Are they important at all? In my interviews and long-term friendships with doctors I find the most prevalent "belief system" to be a form of existentialism. For some doctors, medicine *is* their religion. The scientific cornerstones of bio-medical research and daily practice offer a confidence in our expanding knowledge and experience that improve patient care and the general health of the public; or, at least they could. We are who we are in a world that we did not create, but in which we live. Good and evil are random in this world, and we are free to choose who we shall become. Virtue and good works are important goals for a developed life, and they have their rewards in the here and now in our relationships, in our art and science, and in our daily work. This understanding of our lives as limited to what we know and see is a powerful inheritance from the past from many persons who have given us in their writings and their art careful analyses of life as human beings on this planet. For many doctors, what we see in our daily work and living is what there is.

Another aspect of the secularity of many physicians is a reflection on a characteristic of doctors noted above—we are responsible for what we do. In discussing the impact of religious faith on medical practice, doctors are apt to reiterate the theme mentioned earlier: we cannot avoid our responsibilities to our patients and to ourselves. There is no God who forgives us our errors and misjudgments. We live with who we are and what we do in medicine as in the rest of our lives. With some doctors, this attitude borders on a cynicism toward tragedy and suffering. When one reviews the overall human venture as if from another planet, there is little evidence of goodness either from a creator or from each other. A tour of duty in the emergency room of an inner-city hospital enlightens one about our society. Cynicism can easily become an informed and reliable description of life.

With this turning aside from formal belief in a God of love, justice, and mercy we also hear reference to religious talk as jargon left over from childhood. The daily experiences of physicians raise serious questions for many about classical interpretations of our life and our fate. Life is seen as a cosmic accident—existential in character—that we struggle to understand and live out as honestly as we can, knowing that our control is negligible, and the promises for the future are from a bygone era. There is no question in the minds of many that "what we see is what there is." History is important, though, and we must not forget traditions that have framed the lives of our forebears. A number of doctors have told me the importance of the ethical and the cultural bases of the faiths their parents professed. Jewish physicians recount with pleasure the family gatherings during holy days when the ancient rituals are carried out. But it is the ethics, the behavioral imperatives of the religion, not the belief in God or scripture, that informs their understanding of their lives and their work. Santa Claus embodies for many the significance of Christmas. A physician raised as a Christian recounted the pleasure of attending church on Sunday, listening to the choir sing, and hearing those old and familiar readings from the Bible that recalled childhood. As the sermon began, the mind wandered off to consider other, more important parts of life. Again, the memory, the informed ethic, and the presence of a community of like-minded persons were the support sought for living out the good life. The secular, not the religious, inheritance of the major religions seems to be the residual that supports many of us.

A geneticist placed the questions very clearly. "What kind of a God—a God of love who is all-knowing, all-powerful, and present everywhere—what kind of a God would allow the genetic catastrophes we see? Can there be a God of love who—creator and sustainer of all—is the cause of what we, as physicians, see in this world?" These questions cannot be answered easily; perhaps not at all. But they do raise issues that are serious concerns of patients and may need to be discussed as they face the crises of serious disease and questions about their immediate fate. If physicians have some understanding of faith issues and concerns, they can assist their patients in finding resources for strength and knowledge without compromising the foundations for their own inner life.

Differing Responses

Doctors differ greatly in their responses to caring for the very sick, for those who are dying, and for those for whom further treatment appears to be futile. It is a common observation by patients that physicians often have difficulty discussing dying and death. A variety of reasons are offered for their reluctance to talk about death and to provide the consistent and compassionate care that patients require as death becomes an approaching reality. There have been a few small studies that suggest that some persons are attracted to medicine as a career because they have an undue fear of death and suffering, surpassing that of run-of-the-mill citizens. We may well be attracted to literature, to films and plays, and perhaps even to our specific profession or area of expertise because they express, in one way or another, very basic needs we have for understanding ourselves. Since our subconscious life is just that—below our ordinary discernment—we may not be aware of the reasons for all that we do. There could be some truth to that assertion for we know that persons are often drawn to events and to relationships that hold a fascination or a revulsion for them.

Others have suggested that there is a quasi-belief, a form of magical thinking, held by some persons that, if they become physicians, they will be able to prevent, or at least forestall, their own death. The profession becomes the vehicle for living as long as possible, perhaps even avoiding death. These hypotheses are interesting, and may contain a grain of truth; it is correct that many physicians have great difficulty caring for the dying, for breaking bad news, for being with—and for—the very sick. Another, more plausible, reason for the commonly noted difficulties some doctors have in attending dying patients is the unfortunate idea that physicians care for the living, not the dying. When death is imminent there is little that a doctor can do. Death is understood as the enemy who has won the battle, and the doctor retires from the fray honorably, leaving the care of the patient to others—nurses, chaplains, and social workers. The dying patient is an obvious example of the failure to elicit a cure, the result hoped for, even if not a rational expectation. The goal of the physician is preservation of life; when that is no longer a possibility, the doctor is no longer needed. A bothersome and sad observation of medical sociologists confirms the observation that doctor visits become briefer as the patient gets sicker, often diminishing to simply poking the head in the room and asking, "Hello, how are you today?"

In addition to the arguments offered above for distancing behavior on the part of those whom we trust to care for us when we are gravely ill, there are others we must consider when the medical outcome is doubtful at best. It is not that doctors are less sensitive than others to the needs we have at times of sickness; there is no inevitable characteristic of doctors that predisposes them to this behavior. Most of us are not comfortable in these situations, even with family members and intimate friends; being with—caring for—someone who is suffering, perhaps in pain and frightened, is not an easy task. But, with those close to us, affection and love can conquer anxiety and help us cope. We may not have much expertise in caring for very sick persons, but we do what we can, learning as we go along because there are powerful reasons for doing so: gratitude, love, sympathy, honor, even duty owed to those who cared for us in the past.

The disengagement from feelings, occurring both in medical students and in doctors, is another way of dealing with the internalization of the pressures of caring for seriously ill patients. As noted above, this is a common means of controlling the tensions of practice and the direct management of the painful and emotional issues that arise. A man with widely metastatic pancreatic cancer, for whom his physicians could offer no hope of cure, declined chemotherapy and decided to go home and live out the balance of his life there with family and friends. This decision was accepted by his family; he was an emotionally stable and thoughtful man, one whom the staff thought would "die well." As they were preparing to leave the hospital, his wife spoke to the doctor, explaining that this would be a new, unsettling, and anxiety-producing experience for her. Did the doctor have any suggestions for her when the disease had progressed and her husband became very sick? The doctor looked at her, thought for a moment, and replied, "You can always dial 911." It is difficult to imagine a more terrifying scenario than that, one more devoid of feelings of sympathy and compassion.

At the other end of the spectrum are those who, for reasons of their own, become involved with the personal lives of their patients to the detriment of all. The extreme example is sexual intimacy between patient and doctor, a disastrous situation for the patient; a moral and professional failure for the physician. As with the doctor of 911 fame, behavior is an expression of interior needs, beliefs, and interpretations of the role of the doctor. A hope for all of us is that physicians can be trained to be with and for their patients without going to either extreme of abandonment or intimacy. We shall look later at ways that patients can teach doctors appropriate ways to care for the very sick.

One of the basic beliefs that I hear physicians and surgeons recount after discussing years of experience with its rewards, challenges, and revelations is a certain confidence that *we* give our life its meaning. Through our work, our relationships, our promises and commitments, we determine who we are. We practice our profession to the best of our abilities, in full knowledge of our potential for failure and error. We ask for time to reflect upon our lives and our work, we recognize our need for ongoing study and training to maintain our skills, and we hope that we shall continue to serve the sick and the suffering. But with all this, there remains a need to enrich the life, grasp the day-to-day experiences, and become the doctors we hope to be. Some of our best teachers in this search will be the patients in our care, many of whom know very well their needs, their strengths, and their hopes that reside in confidence in their doctors.

3

"How Do I Do This?"

Hey, Doctor Mermann, I thought this was supposed to be a course
on death and dying; all my patient wants to talk about is living and
getting on with her life!

How can medical students learn to become compassionate physicians, sensitive to the intensely private concerns of others who
are very sick? How will they prevent their potential lapse into the
negative professional traits they will see in their future teachers:
avoidance of the seriously ill and an unfortunate and all-too-apparent
inability to talk about personal issues? Will the intense and interior
questions about life and death, pain and suffering, hope and despair
that patients have—so sharply focused by the intensity of their personal ordeals—prove to be overwhelming and unanswerable? These
questions are important, not only to the students, but also to the faculty that teach our future doctors. Even more significantly, they are
crucial questions for persons who become patients. We expect, or at
least hope for, competence in the professional skills of our doctors,
although this is not always the case.

In the realms of interpersonal reactions, communication competence, and sensitivity to personal and private needs and feelings, there is a wide range of capabilities among physicians. There are significant and visible differences in personalities and their expression in relationships; there are also differences in education and in training of doctors that are factors as they talk with patients and learn their concerns and needs. Patients present themselves with problems, not with diseases. They have symptoms and signs, and concerns and fears, that they hope the physician will make sense of and interpret in an understandable way. Ray Fitzpatrick, lecturer in medical sociology at the University of London, writes,

> The clinician's task is not only to arrive at a diagnosis of the diseases in terms of abnormal physical or mental functioning (and in many instances no disease can be found) but also to identify the illness— the concerns and perceptions that organize and motivate the patient's consultation.[1]

How do we learn? There are many pathways to knowledge and all have roles in our education. Certainly, the road to learning best known to students is attending lectures. In our academic world, lectures by course instructors are the most common way of presenting not only factual information, but controversial issues, ideas, and concepts. Often, indeed, notes are handed out that duplicate the material presented by the lecturer. There is enough history behind this technique to support its ongoing use, but it is not the only, or best, way to teach. Again, in colleges and universities, students advance to learning in small groups—seminars—and, finally, a fortunate student may have an advisor, a mentor, who teaches one-on-one. In an attempt to teach compassionate care, the intricacies of physician-patient interactions, and the complicated individual needs we have when we become sicker and may be dying, a lecture presentation with notes and a reading list can be an inadequate and dull way to teach students. A parallel example could be a lecture by a celibate hermit to an auditorium filled with newlyweds on the nature of human love in its many guises, and the complexities, delights, and frustrations of parenting. The listeners are being taught by one who has read the pertinent literature, attended weddings, perhaps even baptized babies; the only missing factors are being married and a parent. So, too, in the intense and personal area of care of the seriously ill and dying patients, the lecture format is an educational tool that is once-removed from the reality of the need.

I have offered an elective course at the Yale University School of Medicine for first-year medical students—the Seminar on the Seriously Ill Patient—since 1986. The core of the course is the use of patients as teachers of the students. It is important to understand this emphasis, so different from most teaching and formal education in colleges and graduate schools in the United States. We are well aware of public interest in the care offered—medical, social, financial, and psychological—to those of us who are very sick and approaching the end of life. Legal cases and conferences on medical ethics are sharply focused upon issues of autonomy, physician-assisted suicide, euthanasia, advanced directives, living wills, and discontinuing treatment of dying patients. Because of this public and professional interest and concern, many medical schools include lectures on "death and dying" in courses that focus on the role of the doctor in caring for these patients.

However, most of us know, in our personal lives, that we often learn best by *doing,* by participating in the process, by trying it out, by helping an expert in the job at hand. There is, in fact, a common saying about learning medical procedures: "See one, do one, teach one!" This saying may well make some patients nervous, and it is a bit of an exaggeration; but, like "practice makes perfect," it suggests that we learn best by doing, by participation in the event. One of the most respected methods of participation in the learning process with a knowledgeable teacher is that of dialogue, of questioning and discussing the known facts, the possibilities and the probabilities, and the experiences of others in similar situations. Certainly, in the practice of medicine, it is essential to get the story straight; the interviewer must look for inconsistencies, telltale hints, errors in understanding, and misinterpretations of events that could lead to faulty reasoning.

The most famous of all questioning teachers is Socrates, the

Greek philosopher who lived in the fifth century B.C.E., for whom questioning was central to learning. What we can know of the Good and of virtue lies within us; by questioning and analyzing we can learn the way we are to go in this life, how we are to be with and for others, what behaviors will define us to ourselves and to the world. The good teacher is defined by commitment to the role of instructor, and is possessed by that urgent desire to help others learn what must be known, and a deep confidence in the ability of the student to learn essential facts that are then transmuted into new knowledge and new expectations. This method is an ongoing process and the hope is, of course, that the student will become wise in learning and skilled in the craft of the profession, carrying on the great tradition of teaching by experience.

The basic technique—Socratic dialogue—as the teaching tool in our learning is based upon a strong conviction that we already have the knowledge we need for living our lives in an honorable fashion. The facts can be gathered and memorized; it is the reasoned and thought-through living that is so important. Within us are the possibilities for life behavior that is exemplary. Defining characteristics of human excellence such as justice and mercy, compassion and sensitivity, honesty and goodness: these are integral to us as persons. The teacher takes on, as Socrates suggested, the role of a midwife who assists in the delivery of these virtues. We are taught to realize that they are essential to us and to our self-defining behavior, and we must find them within our personalities so that we will behave in ways that honor us and our work. As an instructor, I do not teach you to tell the truth, as if that idea were foreign to you; I do not tell you that you should be kind to others, as if you had never thought of that. No; by ongoing and serious *dialogue*—not lecture—you and I learn that the impulses to honorable and caring behavior have always been within us. With an educational method leading to self-understanding and awareness, we realize that we are able to live the life we had barely imagined as possible.

There are other aspects to this teaching method that are central to its importance for students learning to care for seriously ill persons: the teacher is also a student, a learner in the ongoing dialogue. The patient does not merely teach the student what it is like to be sick, take medications, worry, and fear the future. The patient is also learning—by teaching—the strengths and the possibilities that are within us for living an honorable life and dying an admirable death. In teaching about human experiences we can learn about ourselves; we can have revelations about meaning and value, commitment and relationships that inform us further than we anticipated. These concerns are important to all patients, but, again, not limited to them; they are central to the comprehended self of all caregivers in whatever profession or role. One of the universal experiences of teachers is that we probably learn more in the process of teaching than do the students. After all, the hope we hold for ourselves is that we can learn to live a good life in relationships with others and in harmony with what we know of ourselves. Whether we are patient or caregiver is a question of this moment only; we shall all assume the role of patient, dress for the part, and act out that character in the drama of our future time. The goal of this Socratic method of learning is that teacher and student are both learning the lessons of life, the hopes we hold together on this common journey, and our responsibilities to—and for—each other.

I intentionally offer this seminar to first-year students. It might seem more plausible to do this type of teaching during their third year, that concentrated time of learning the diagnostic and therapeutic function of the profession in the hospital, specialty outpatient clinics, and the offices of physicians who teach the intricacies of patient care. However, by the time students are doing clinical work, their focus, and their instructors' interests, lie in the clinical work. This can leave little time for the personal, nonscientific components of the life of the patient. First-year students, in contrast, know no medicine; they have just arrived in school and are increasing their necessary knowledge of the basic biological nature of our bodies before they go on to learn of diseases, and diagnostic and treatment techniques.

The medical students approach this seminar with some anxiety. Many of them present a most engaging paradox: they want to learn how to talk with sick persons in a meaningful and sympathetic way, yet they are quite nervous about the methods we use to communicate with others. "How do I do this?" is a common question asked during the first two or three meetings I have with the students at the beginning of the semester. In anticipation of the question, I focus our first two sessions on talk about the content of our conversations with persons we do not know well; how we initiate a conversation with a stranger, particularly in the situation where one is unwell, the setting is unfamiliar, and the topic a most serious one. The students, quite understandably, feel nervous about their first encounter with their patient-teachers. For many students, the academic focus upon physical sciences in secondary school and college precludes a developed social life. The competition for matriculation in medical schools is impressive, and grades in courses are significant qualifiers for acceptance. This may, for some students, limit the amount of time and energy they have invested in developing their skills in serious conversation about their personal concerns.

On the other side of the dialogue that I hope to establish are patients who are unwell, receiving chemotherapy or other debilitating treatments and procedures that weaken and depress them. Their concerns about their disease are all-encompassing: its progress or retreat, and the uncertainties of the future. The effects of serious disease extend beyond the patient to include others for whom responsibility continues, for intimate relationships and friendships of long standing, and to matters of spirit that determine our selves. All of these can present severe limitations on casual conversation.

Learning the skills of interviewing is so important for establishing a secure professional link between patient and doctor. James Thompson, lecturer in psychology at the University of London, writes,

> Despite being the cornerstone of medical practice, [the interview] is often seen as a tiresome interface between the doctor and the disease, yet it may determine the form and content of the information provided, and may totally determine whether the advice given is heeded. . . . [D]issatisfaction with medical communications remain the most prominent of patient complaints and a major factor in the

move to alternative medicine, with its focus on good and reassuring communications and the patient as an informed participant in treatment. Patients prefer to be able to give an account of their problems in their own terms, yet these expectations of communication are often unmet.[2]

Certainly, patient compliance with advice on treatments, changes in lifestyle, and with follow-up visits is strongly influenced by the relationship established so quickly during the initial interview. Bringing together an anxious student and a patient sharply focused upon the self is an impressive challenge for creating a teaching and learning dialogue between strangers. The challenge is met quite easily, to the surprise of many. Its resolution lies in the commitments of both the students and the patients to goals that lie distinctly outside the personal needs of each. The students bring their professional hopes for becoming physicians committed to compassionate care of future patients. The patients are equally committed, but to the task of teaching. The mild insecurity that students experience places them, early in their careers, in a position without the power they will have after training. They attend to their assigned patient-teacher without having any agenda of their own in terms of time or predetermined ideas about the patient's disease, personal life, emotional state, or medical expertise. They are merely attentive to being taught what it means to be sick. One student, writing about his patient-teacher, says,

> I can describe her as a teacher in both the literal and figurative sense of the word. She taught math in a local middle school until she was diagnosed with ovarian cancer about two years ago, which had gone into remission and then spread to her small intestine. But when I met her in the fall, she was very optimistic and open, feeling that her new round of chemotherapy could help her and that she wanted to help me, as a first-year student, to understand what patients go through when seriously ill. From the moment I met her, she told me everything, her sadness at having lost both of her parents recently to cancer, her hope that she wouldn't meet the same fate, her fears at what her family would do without her, and her desire to

keep faith in this time of trouble. I couldn't imagine being so open with a literal stranger. But to her, it was simply an exercise in teaching, perhaps a final metaphor for a career she must have done extremely well.[3]

This is not a new task for many older persons. So many adults—as parents, grandparents, volunteers in service organizations, teachers, religious believers, or political activists—are committed to conveying to the coming generations their values and the fundamental needs we have to live in community. The patients whom I recruit for the seminar almost universally agree to be teachers, invariably acknowledging quite openly their awareness of the need for physicians to learn the basic skills of communication, sympathy, and companionship during their coming journey. They know the need exists.

Occasionally, in talking with a prospective patient-teacher, there is some hesitation on the part of the patient. Will the proposed ongoing dialogue with the student interfere with appointments and treatments? Will the time spent with the student mean an undesired prolonged stay in the clinic? Will the patient be exhausted—physically and emotionally—by discussing intimate personal issues? Will insensitive and embarrassing questions be asked? I assure patients that the conversations are controlled by them in content, form, and duration; I and the students are grateful for the time spent, the concerns discussed, and the personal, often intimate, information shared. When patients are still hesitant, I rely upon my ultimately irresistible argument. Talking with first-year medical students about these topics will give patients an opportunity to teach neophyte students, from their own experiences, the differences between a good doctor and a "not-so-good doctor." Very few patients can stay away from that baited hook; they have had experiences they are all quick to relate, and with considerable feeling. These are experiences from which we all can learn the appropriate care of patients.

In preparing the students for their encounters with their patient-teachers we watch some videos on how doctors and patients talk—or do not talk—with each other, and an unedited film of an interview with a dying patient that provides ample opportunities for comment and enlightenment. But the main burden of the teaching is in the hands of the patients with whom I have discussed the purposes of the seminar, and the ways by which they can inform students about the essentials of good medical care. This material is carefully described in an information sheet the patients receive. Strict confidentiality is enforced as students learn that their patient-teachers cannot be referred to by name: physicians must never speak of patients in ways that identification by others is possible. I point out to the patients the likely apprehension of the students, commenting on the polarity the patients will note: a real and clearly stated desire to learn, balanced by anxiety around the experience of talking about serious personal concerns. The students are nervous about intruding on the inner territory of the lives of their patient-teachers; but, at the same time they want to learn how to gain the confidence of their teachers so that they will know what happens to us when we are very sick. They will also learn what patients expect from a good doctor. As one would anticipate, the patient-teachers are usually fully equipped to bring their students along the path of learning. After all, they do speak from exquisitely personal experiences.

There is an impressive variety of patient-teachers, as one would expect. There is no perfect one, since we are as unique in our personalities as we are in our bodies. This is an important fact for the students to understand. In small-group discussions each week the students present their ongoing sagas of their encounters with their teachers. This seminar offers the proving ground for learning the varied methods of dealing with serious disease. Each student relates different stories which, when assembled, offer the students a new and documented understanding of our profound differences. The students learn that there is no single way to deal with the exigencies of serious illness; some coping techniques seem more effective than others, but this is open to individual interpretation. In this process of recounting their dialogues with their teachers and comparing notes on the varied ways we confront crises, the students learn what to expect in their future careers, and how to gather and assimilate this precious personal patient experience. In a sense, in the small groups each student has the opportunity to learn from the other patients and students; it is like talking to the ultimate patient, one who has all the diseases, describes the manifold ways we react to those diseases, and therefore presents the qualities of the caring physician, that eagerly, if somewhat anxiously, hoped-for goal of students. A human trait that a patient awaits expectantly from a physician is sympathy for their experience with their disease. In the small-group conversations we make an effort to identify with the responses that the patients, their spouses and children, and their friends and co-workers make to the disease and its impact on life. In most of our relationships, a sense of a sympathetic ear listening to our story, even if nothing can be done to change the course of events, is a most welcome event.

Another goal that I set for students is learning that we can talk with patients about those very personal issues that fluster us at first because they are so delicate. But these personal notes do determine us, and help the student learn that being a person is quite a spectacular event. To encourage an open discussion of the many—often polarized—feelings patients have in their stressful hours is a visible sign of our commitment to them. A student captures, in a fiction derived from her conversations with her patient-teacher, this autobiographical sketch:

> My identity has been reduced to Patient, on this page and in my life. And yet another day you might have bumped into me in the street, caught sight of me over bunches of asparagus at the supermarket, or received the plate from me on a Sunday morning. Our eyes would have met, we would have smiled, you might have wanted to kiss me or confide in me. But no one falls in love with a cancer patient. I'm sexless, devoid of vitality. Each morning, out of habit, I pick out my clothes with care; most things hang strangely on my newly svelte figure, and dark colors make me look shockingly pale. But then I stop and wonder, "Why do I even bother? What does it matter, at this point?" My friends have either disappeared or have taken to smothering me with kindness. New acquaintances retreat, awkwardly.[4]

For medical students hoping to become good doctors, patients are superb teachers of the skills known collectively as "bedside manners."

There is a sentimental, yet serious, note to that word *manners*: it implies politeness and a willing exchange of information and opinion; courteousness, and acknowledgment of rights, privileges, and responsibilities; also a careful delineation of the personal limits so essential for dedicated and attentive care. In all our relationships— from marriage to psychotherapy to a card game—we need to know our responsibilities, fulfill our promises, and do our dedicated work, all within carefully outlined and recognized boundaries. Having a serious, perhaps life-threatening, disease certainly engages the whole rainbow of feelings that we can know. Sensitivity to this fact, and willingness to discuss the associated anxieties, fears, and complicated decisions that must be made, are key parts to the support the caring physician provides. To deny that these feelings exist is to undervalue the humanity of the patient, admitting, by example, that the physician either does not know of them or considers them of little import.

Another aspect of learning to talk with patients about their lives is truly paying attention to what is being said, looking for inconsistencies, incoherent reciting of symptoms, and confusion about detail. Without being offensive, the good interviewer will help the patient clarify the true nature of the events, the feelings, and the responses that led up to the present state. When done with care, the interview can establish a powerful bond that will ensure ongoing cooperation. It is a fine compliment to our patients when we acknowledge that the emotional side of our lives is also defining who we are. A student for whom an ended relationship caused a deep sense of loss learned from her patient-teacher that life goes on.

> A relationship begins. . . . I walk into a room streaked with sunlight and see a woman lying in bed. She quickly puts on her hat to hide her scalp which is bare from chemotherapy. She has acute myelogenous leukemia. She was a librarian until a year and a half ago when she began to feel extremely tired. I, too, feel extremely tired. But how dare I compare my own tragedy to the pain which threatens her life on a daily basis? Perhaps at this point, I hope somehow that knowing her will give me insights on my loss and take away my sadness. . . .
>
> We do not talk about her death but we talk about her life. We

talk about her illness and her treatment. I imagine the experience of waking up one day and having leukemia. . . . She has a serious illness, but when I see her I do not think of her illness. I see right through the platelets, the tubes, and the whole blood to the woman I have grown to love. . . . She is human. I am human. Illness does not take away her humanity. . . . A serious illness is not simply a prelude to death. A serious illness is a new way of life. In health and in illness, friendships make all the difference.[5]

Willingness to discuss the powerful interior lives we own can be a lasting bond between patient and caregiver. It is a strong compliment to the commonality of human experience to encourage patients and families to speak of their innermost, sometimes conflicted, feelings.

Many of us have difficulty putting our feelings into words and speaking of them with others. Privacy is a condition of our lives not easily set aside, but it is often helpful to be permitted to speak to our feelings since they play such an important part in our everyday living. All of our relationships have feelings tied to them, for good or ill. Students can learn to talk together with patients about our emotional responses to events in our lives that are important; the patient is the teacher for us in this important task. One important qualification must be mentioned: students are taught to speak sparingly of themselves. The purpose of speaking in depth with patients is to further their welfare by learning of their needs and their inner concerns, not to chitchat and compare notes about the details of day-to-day living. In these conversations students learn to recognize emotions in others, evaluate their importance in providing appropriate care, and plan for support and encouragement when the events of our lives run counter to our hopes and expectations.

Openness to the emotions of a patient is a gift to that person. Students can learn the varied way that we send a signal to others that we care, that we are interested in their whole life, not just the disease and its treatments. There are many simple ways to engage another person in a conversation focused upon the significant individuality of that person, and these can be learned and practiced. Questions about the photographs on the bedside table, the book that was being read before this interruption, the personal and social calibre of the characters in the soap opera on the television screen—all these lead easily to talk about personal values, about a life lived this way rather than that way. As this type of speaking together develops over time, students learn to be alert to the casual statement that begs for a question, the offhand comment that suggests that there is much more waiting to be discovered by an inquiring heart and mind. Recognition of the wholeness of the person in our care, attention to the many sides of human personality, a willingness to listen, and an obvious pleasure in knowing a patient as a person can open the doors to a rewarding lifetime of caring for others.

Another surprise in our learning from our patients is a sense of identification with them as persons quite similar to us in their innate and unique personhood, if different in the external vagaries of human existence. As we identify with others, we usually find that our negative judgments of them recede before our acceptance of our sameness in times of joy, sorrow, anxiety, and pain. This new ability to be with and for another without concern for some of the idiosyncratic qualities we all exhibit is a gift we receive from those in our care. Our patients become our teachers in many and varied ways, allowing us to grow and mature in this new way.

Notes

1. R. Fitzpatrick, "Lay Concepts of Illness," *The Experience of Illness* (London: Tavistock Publications, 1984), 27.

2. J. Thompson, "Communicating with Patients," in *The Experience of Illness*, 87.

3. A. Venkut, personal communication, 1996.

4. E. Choo, personal communication, 1996.

5. E. Harrold, personal communication, 1997.

4

Who Suffers?

Suffering is permanent, obscure and dark,
And shares the nature of infinity.
William Wordsworth, *The Borderers*

The ancient and time-honored function, indeed, the duty, of the physician is relief of pain and suffering. These two words, *pain* and *suffering*, are so often spoken and written together that it is almost as if they were one. If not quite recognized as one word, they are understood by many as closely related, the first causing the second. But I do not think that this is always true. Pain relief is a traditional expectation we have of the doctor; access to narcotics and other medications should guarantee that patients will not have to manage their pain by themselves. Many physicians fail to use their knowledge and training to care properly for their patients in pain. The Hospice movement was begun in England as an innovative response to the suffering of persons dying without proper attention to their pain. Suffering caused by pain should, in most instances, be relieved by prompt and proper medical management. There are always exceptions to any rule, of course, and suffering and pain can certainly be intimately associated, particularly in chronic diseases such as arthritis, diabetes, and certain gastrointestinal disorders that can plague us for years.

Suffering is a difficult word to define, in part because suffering is such a personal response that we have to events in our lives. These may, or may not, be related to medical problems. Certainly the death of someone loved, destruction of a cherished creation we brought into being, revealed deception by a trusted friend—all these can cause suffering beyond the possibility of relief by a doctor. We will look to these universal causes of suffering later. It may well be true that less suffering is known to us because of disease and accidents than by the losses we experience as members of families and communities, the failures we must accept as ours, and the questionable morality of some of the decisions we have made. But there are many medical causes for suffering: diseases that cause us misery and anguish, fear and resentment, despair and anger beyond the confines of the disease itself.

But first, what is it that we call suffering? The relief of suffering is such an accepted expectation that patients have of their doctors that we need a common language to discuss it. The impact of the suffering of patients on the physician is often considerable and impressive in both professional and personal ways. Feelings of insecurity and incompetence before the magnitude of the suffering of others can be nearly overwhelming, and a source of distress. A well-known and respected writer on suffering is Eric J. Cassell, M.D., who writes, "I believe suffering to be the distress brought about by the actual or perceived impending threat to the integrity or continued existence of the whole person."[1] He qualifies the phrase *whole person* by including social, psychological, and personal aspects of our lives that define us to ourselves and to others.

The broadness of his definition allows us to consider the wide potential impact of suffering on the person. The possibilities for suffering are important because the fears and the anxieties we have about suffering relate primarily to the future; we are afraid of the suffering we may have to endure. We seem able to get through this moment, but it is the possibility of unbearable pain or misery or self-disgust that might lie ahead that weighs us down so heavily.

A quality of the sufferer important in our understanding of suffering is endurance. To suffer is to bear a burden, to carry oneself through pain and misery, to hold the self together through experiences that are damaging, destructive, and demeaning to us as persons in our world, the existence we know and claim as our own. There are so many stories of persons who have held on when all hope seemed gone: hikers and explorers, parents and children, friends who would not leave their afflicted companions, nurses and doctors who stay when there seems little expectation for recovery. I consider endurance to be an ultimate virtue in understanding the meanings that suffering holds for us. For we will all suffer at one time or another in our lives. Central to the purposes of this study is enhancing the role of the physician in alleviating suffering, finding effective and reliable means to teach medical students the significance and the power of suffering in our lives, and the hopes we have for knowing the valued companionship of the compassionate physician who has learned from patients the needs of the sufferer.

There are many ways in which we suffer, as there are also many reasons for our suffering. Just as all suffering does not have a physical cause, so understanding and management of suffering is not restricted to medications and treatments. A common form of suffering—almost laughable at times—is the anxiety patients have during hospitalization. There are the obvious major questions about diagnosis and treatment. But there are also disruption of daily habits, the wearing of odd clothing, a schedule that seems to make little sense, and the basic question of outcome. Reassurance in this environment can be supportive. Social class plays a role here because economic factors are important in what we are forced to endure. If seeking medical care involves time lost from work, difficulty getting to the medical facility, and impersonal care after arriving, persons will often suffer with their diseases, accepting them as a fatalistic occurrence. Also, social class can be a determinant of a decision about what constitutes sickness. If paying rent and putting food on the table are daily questions, certain sets of signs and symptoms may be ignored as common to our lot and not an emergency. For some, the emergency department at the hospital is the family doctor, whose help is sought for medical and social problems no longer bearable.

If physicians are to be alert to those who suffer, they must learn of these other forms of suffering from their patients. There are many causes of the distresses that damage and isolate us from others in our worlds that must be endured. I make an arbitrary division of suffering into the three classical modes of understanding the parts of us that have traditionally defined us as human beings: body, mind, and spirit. This is a construct for learning and for teaching; obviously we are whole persons and there is no way to actually divide us into parts. I am a body going about my business in the world, acting and reacting, thinking and feeling, in wonder and awe, not a person divided, like Caesar's Gaul, into three parts. But this classical division of ourselves as persons offers a structure for learning about suffering and the means by which physicians can act responsibly toward those confident in their care.

We are whole persons, yet in a way like a puzzle with many pieces that must be placed together properly if we are to recognize the picture, acknowledging others as individuals, as entities like ourselves. We are each unique in our inherited chromosomes and genes; with the exception of identical twins, and the distinct future possibilities of cloning, no other person is the same as each of us. This is important to keep in mind since our responses to similar events can be widely different. As Ellen Glasgow wrote somewhere, "a laceration to one is an amputation to another." We are not the same as another, and we will not respond the same way to nearly identical situations, diseases, desires, or pleasures. But we do understand ourselves in similar ways: we recognize our bodies as being constructed in ways consonant to others, and we know our emotions that encompass such different feelings as anxiety and affection are common to us. There is yet another part of us that responds, perhaps fitfully and unwillingly, to a recurring deep search for the meanings of life, a reverence for the awe we know in this infinite universe beyond our comprehension: our life in the spirit. Each of these parts of what we know to be a person—here artificially separated for the purpose of learning compassionate care for the needs of others—can most certainly suffer. But before I discuss the experiences of suffering I will present various aspects of our lives, parts of what we know of ourselves that makes us knowable as persons, that unique amalgam of body, mind, and spirit combined into a whole piece of cloth from our very beginning.

What Is a Person?

Each one of us, regardless of our physical, emotional, and intellectual capabilities, is a person. We have a very large set of defining characteristics that tells others, as well as ourselves, who we are. Most of us have extraordinary gifts to give. Most of us, also, are limited in some of varied capacities. No one can lay claim to perfection. But we know that we are to recognize one and all as persons deserving of respect and capable of suffering, although perhaps not in ways that we would recognize. The various components of being a person that I will review do determine how we respond to the distinguishing events of our lives: marriage, parenting, work, play, friendships, and—especially—to our suffering and our dying. But we are not strictly determined or limited by a certain personality, by inherited and cultural specifics, and by our bodies, and must therefore behave in certain ways without the possibilities for change. What is important is that we recognize who we are, and how we respond to our many-faceted world; this will enable us to recognize the possibilities for change, and for growth and maturation that enable us to understand by anticipation and preparation the problems that lie ahead. There will be suffering and loss, pain and despair in the future; knowing who we are and the resources we have at our disposal will improve our competence in coping with suffering. There is a clear need for us to learn how to know ourselves, to grasp the particularities of our own persons, as we prepare for our future with its uncertainties and its inevitabilities.

As persons we have a past, that accumulation of experiences and events, of memories of joy and sadness, of hopes realized and destroyed that tell us who we are today. This unique past has its effects on each day's decisions, hopes, and acts. We have traveled a road unique to us and we are now at a specific point in our lives where our responses are determined by that past. Our past includes an education, formal or otherwise, that we use now to interpret what is happening to and around us. That education may inform us, it may prejudice us, it may misinform us, but it has its effect. We begin each day carrying with us our singular and exclusive baggage of experiences that will color each happening of the day, be it good, bad, or indifferent. Reflection on our past is essential for coping with the stresses of our lives, particularly as we face disease and the suffering that will accompany it. It is so important to avoid a "knee-jerk" response to a diagnosis that suggests serious consequences by assuming either the worst and giving up, or counting on a miracle to eliminate the problem. We must look within our selves, evaluating events according to our remembered past, and plan our future accordingly.

Our past experiences are the stage setting for the drama that is unfolding. We are onstage, the curtain is rising, and the play is about to begin. All of our experiences with sickness, medical-care providers, pain, loneliness and companionship, assurances and fears will come to bear on the responses we make to illness. We know of family members, friends, acquaintances, even movie stars who have been sick and had various outcomes. We have had, or have heard of diseases, disabilities, treatments, and unexpected encounters with physicians and surgeons. Which will be ours? We have read of this and that experience of others, and we have matched them against our own. We have been with others who have suffered, and wondered about how we might react to the same event if and when it happened to us. And now here we are, calling up those experiences to help us this very day with our own confrontation with illness.

Another crucial determinant of being a person is the relationships we have with others, those ties that define so much of the world we know and, often quite unknowingly, so clearly determine our responses to experience. Family plays a major role in our lives, having profound effects on us long before we are even aware of them. There are so many places in which we fit, so many roles we play. The effects on us and others of being a father or mother, a sister or brother are permanent and powerful. Expectations placed upon us by our culture, by our position in the hierarchy of the family, and by our own wishes to fulfill our role fully are heavy burdens for many to carry. One could say that, from the moment of conception, family is a powerful influence on us in establishing a protective or alienating environment, setting standards and demands that can never be met, and revealing ways of giving and receiving, of promising and deceiving that lay out the future of the child not yet born.

Certainly the centuries of abuse of children—continuing well into our own times—show how profound disastrous family relationships are determinants of our behavior in the face of potential catastrophe. Only in recent years has the long history of child abuse been presented so clearly to us. The damage remains a significant and defining part of the life of the child into adulthood, altering and corrupting the relationships hoped for in life. Whether this type of damage can be repaired remains a question for many. How we interpret what is, has, and will happen to us is intimately tied to how we have been raised from the moment of our birth, if not, as suggested, from our conception.

A related determinant of what it means to be a person is the effect of the roles we play in our lives. We each play these roles over and over again each day. We are worker, parent, spouse, citizen, member of varied and disparate groups with others. These roles are very defining, by the world around us if not always by ourselves. An intricate and enveloping web is woven by our very living in society. Others have expectations of us in each role that we play; we must know what these expectations are so that we can fulfill them and meet the demands that confront us each moment. How we understand the different—often conflicting—roles we are called upon to play will tell others who we are, and will determine how we shall respond to the crises in our lives, the inevitable roadblocks, if not final stopping places, that are human experiences. We are beset by the conflicts we have. As a member of our common human community I am appalled by documented reports of hunger, deprivation, and killing that abound on the earth. The number of persons without access to health care is a disgrace to the expectations I have for my own behavior as a citizen and as a physician. The epitome of religious response to obvious need, in so many traditions, is generosity shown to the poor even if that entails sacrifice. Do I, as laid out so clearly by Jesus in his conversation with the rich young man, give all I have to the poor and follow him? What then, of the needs of my family, my old age, my simple pleasures? Our roles place us in conflict, not only with our society, but with ourselves. When crises erupt, decisions can be confounded, clarified, distorted, or defined by our roles.

As persons we are influenced by our cultural background. In sickness these influences are powerful and determine not only our understanding of the causes, characteristics, and treatments of diseases, but also the significance and the meaning of disease for us. We now know the strong influences of diet on causing the pathological changes in our bodies that will prove fatal. Personal behavior with its taking of risks or protecting the self, exposure to harmful environments of many types, and disregard of basic health standards cause disease and disability and can deflect the expected good effects of therapy. How one behaves when ill—the sick role—is often directed by the society in which one lives. A dour Scot will not understand the Latin American categories of disease as "hot" and "cold." Illness, as inevitable punishment for sin—the certain consequence of specific behavior—will be understood by others as a challenge to an enduring faith in a loving God. A physician trained in anatomy in a European or American medical school finds the anatomical basis for acupuncture completely beyond comprehension. Concepts of miracles, consequences of prayer, the meaning of sacrifice—all are examples of accepted understanding of individual universes that sharply determine personal and cultural reactions to serious illness. Having even an elementary knowledge of these facts can be an acknowledged aid in providing compassionate care by accepting the inevitable boundaries and categories that our culture imposes on us.

As persons we have an inner life. This interior existence unknown to others can be a fanciful one of hoped-for successes and accomplishments; it can be a fantastic life of unrealistic expectations and dreams; it can be a firm and defined future for which one trains and plans and sacrifices, hoping to bring into existence a piece of work, a poem, a solution for the despair so many of us know in our everyday lives. The inner life can also be a secret life of relationships that are taboo, of behavior that is banned, of acts that are ostracized. All of these are possible definers of us and will be factors requiring consideration when disease interrupts our lives and brings the future to an alarming halt by introducing the unknown and the unanticipated. For many of us, the future is a time for the realization of our hopes: the bringing to fruition the possible and the potential accomplishments we are capable of performing. It is not that we would remake the world or solve its insoluble problems. It is, rather, that we would live an honorable life of work and relationships, in hope that rewards would be adequate to know that the work was good, the relationships valid and true.

A number of years ago a colleague was diagnosed with an untreatable cancer. In our conversations he offered a superb metaphor for one of the modes of his suffering. Of course, he anticipated pain, but expected that it would be treated; he mourned in advance his pending separation from his family and friends; and he was saddened as he thought about his abbreviated career. He put it poignantly, saying that there would be no second act in his life. At this time when he had been successful in achieving a tenured appointment, when research and writing were progressing well, when competition with others was no longer an issue—at this very moment—his life was ending. The curtain was coming down and the first act was over; there would be no second act. This was a cause for suffering in its many guises indeed.

A significant part of an honorable life of work and relationships will be the expression of our sexuality in trustworthy and enriching ways that show forth our willingness to give as much as we receive, if not more. Throughout history the expression of our sexual nature has been an integral part of our very lives. The perpetuation of our species, as with most others, is dependent upon the mating of female and male. Not only is reproduction a result of our sexual impulses and drives; sexual intercourse can be one of the most profound expressions of devotion between two persons, linking them in a most profound intimacy. One of the more distressing losses suffered by us in sickness is the end of sexual experience. Sexual expression is revealed in a number of ways, both in hetero- and homosexual

modes. Acceptance of our innate differences is essential if we are to
live in community with respect and care for each other. The powerful
grip that sexuality has on us can be an added cause for suffering when
the one we love is a secret to family, friends, and caregivers; sickness
then separates lovers at the time of deepest need.

The definitive characteristic of our sexual lives is caring for one's
partner in ways that express love and respect. Even after the physical
acts of intercourse are no longer possible, intimacy and affection
remain central. One of the first patients I asked to talk with me and
the students about being very sick was a young woman with leukemia
in the last weeks of her life. As she talked about the losses she knew,
she spoke about her intimate life with her husband and their young
children. Pale, weak, and exhausted, she smiled, amazingly, as she
described how every day at lunchtime her husband would come to
the hospital to visit. He came into her room, pulled down the curtain
on the door, and got into the hospital bed with his wife so that they
might hold each other for a few hours and speak of their loves, both
for each other and all the others in their lives. For the students, as for
me, awe and silence were our responses.

One of the aspects of personhood whose loss in sickness is noted
frequently is that odd assortment of acts and behaviors that we might
term daily, or day-by-day duties. So many of us are defined, often significantly, by housekeeping chores, cutting the grass and tending the
garden, shopping, child care, preparing meals for family and friends,
chatting about the events of the day. Few of us will achieve any
prominence in the world out there; fame and fortune—whose eternal
values are questionable at best—will not be achievements many of us
will acquire. Occasionally, as I listen to the music of Mozart or
Vivaldi, I imagine myself in a concert hall in Vienna, or in St. Mark's
in Venice. I look at the women and men seated around me, the
orchestra performing the heavenly music actually composed by the
conductor, and I realize that only the composers will be remembered:
the rest of us will be forgotten, indeed forgotten forever. I frequently
remind myself of this when I recall the old saw "We'll never forget
'what's-his-name'! " And so, for most of us, the daily experiences of
living will tell us and our world who we are in our very persons. Our

suffering will be revealed in the loss of our living out our everyday lives.

If we are to understand the nature of suffering, what it means for others and will mean for us, then we must understand the multiple pieces that go together to make us into persons, the different, yet related, aspects of personhood described above. Central to our study of suffering is, of course, the suffering our bodies will endure, the pain we will bear. This important aspect will be developed in the following chapter. We are each, in our own way, a composite person with a past and a future, with hopes and aspirations, with dreams and nightmares. We are each inheritors of family and of culture, players of roles and livers of relationships. We can each bear the burdens of others, and seek the help of others to bear our own. We do this, each one, with a body, mind, and spirit that we bring to our tasks. We all have experienced parts of life in its plethora of forms, and envied others for what we have never known. But we are persons: we shall certainly suffer, and be called upon to be with and for others who do likewise. The relief of unhappiness, sadness, and despair are our duties. How we do this will, in large part, depend upon how well we know ourselves and how well we are willing to be open to learning from others. This is the task we undertake as we look at the nature of suffering.

How Do We Suffer?

Suffering, that experience to which all persons are open, occurs when we are participants in an event that threatens the wholeness of us, that stretches our understanding of the nature of our lives to a point where meaning and significance begin to pale. Suffering is what we know when our very own personhood is endangered in one or many of the categories noted above. There is a completeness to our person, a sense in which we are what we are, living the life we are living as best we can, "all things considered." When this life is threatened, we suffer. And we suffer in the three component parts of ourselves: body, mind, and spirit. We are to remember that the whole person suffers, not just the body, the mind, or the spirit. I refer to them to highlight the parts of us threatened with dissolution. It is always the person who suffers. We will look at these three parts of ourselves as distinct entities because many of us do see ourselves as so constructed. Also, this will help us see why, in similar circumstances, some persons suffer, and others appear not to show any evidence of it.

A universal form of suffering is being the bearer of a medical or psychological condition stigmatized by others. Throughout our history certain diseases and conditions have carried that burden. Leprosy, in biblical times, was a skin disorder that compelled separation from the community. Epilepsy, blindness, loss of a limb, and deafness are common causes of shunning in our history. Cancer has, for many years, been a diagnosis kept hidden from others. Despite education about, and exposure to, these conditions, persons with them are often marginalized and denied access to public services. Schizophrenia and other mental disorders likewise are causes for alienation. Forms of behavior considered deviant by some are also sources of suffering. Homosexuality continues to be a focus of antagonism and stigmatization in our culture. Sexually transmitted diseases carry the same label. All of these are sources of suffering, and are dealt with by the persons so afflicted in a variety of ways, often by denial and covering up.

The central experience for us as we learn the nature of suffering, its effects upon us in our multiple selves, and the hopes we have for diminishing, if not relieving suffering, is taught us by the sufferers. For medical students and doctors, the teacher is the patient. Who else can inform us of those deep and dark places in ourselves where the suffering sits and haunts? An open mind and heart can bring a new knowledge to the caregiver of the very nature of our humanity. Cassell writes,

> The only way to learn whether suffering is present is to ask the sufferer. We all recognize certain injuries that almost invariably cause suffering: the death or suffering of loved ones, powerlessness, helplessness, hopelessness, torture, the loss of a life's work, deep betrayal, physical agony, isolation, homelessness, memory failure, and unremitting fear. Each is both universal and individual. Each

touches features common to us all, yet each must be defined in terms of a specific person at a specific time.[2]

Notes

1. Eric J. Cassell, "Recognizing Suffering," *Hastings Center Report* 21, no. 3 (May–June 1991): 24.

2. Eric J. Cassell, *The Nature of Suffering* (New York, Oxford University Press, 1991), 44.

5

"I Don't Look in the Mirror"

> Body my house
> my horse my hound
> what will I do
> when you are fallen
>
> May Swenson, *Question* (1954)

I was in the outpatient cancer chemotherapy clinic on Wednesday morning talking with a woman about the seminar, and asked her if she would be interested in teaching a medical student about her experiences. She had had a breast removed several years previously; the cancer recurred and she was in for treatment. As we talked about these past few years and she reflected on her life, she said, "You know, since I had the surgery that removed my breast, I don't look in the mirror anymore. I don't dress in front of it; I can't bear to look at myself." The image I had has stayed with me. I ask myself, "What does a doctor say to this?" What was there to say to her about her response to the violation of her body, necessary though it apparently was? What words can replace a part of our bodies that is such an identifier, such a definer of who we are in our social world? Our understanding of ourselves is so often tied to how we appear to ourselves and to the world. We live in a culture where appearance is a significant determinant of who we are, who we want to be. What I look like tells you who I am. We are so concerned with looking like current models of clothing and accessories. We want to be attractive; a word loaded with meaning in itself. One has only to stand in the checkout line at the supermarket and look at the photographs on the covers of magazines to see the emphasis on youthful, slender, carefully groomed, voluptuous women without a crease or fold anywhere. The men are muscular, tightwaisted, with a full head of hair.

We are obsessed with physical appearance and fitness, concerned more with our appearance and less with our behavior. We are captured by the photographic essays on the best dressed, the worst dressed; we pause at the photos of actresses in their scanty clothes. A sad and worrisome effect of this concern for many women is their conclusion that their bodies are not attractive, that they lack the basic qualities of today's woman, and are, therefore, inadequate in the simplest of ways. This can cause a sad sense of loathing of the self that seems quite beyond the healing power of reassurance, so often manifest in young women with anorexia and bulimia. With aging and its increasing risks of serious disease, there is the real possibility of marked changes in our bodies that will distress us all the more. For many of us, as for the woman I spoke with, what we look like is a major determinant of who we are. It seems a long time ago when we were told, and believed, that beauty was only skin deep. Our bodies play a very large role in our understanding of who we are in our worlds, private and public.

When we become sick, or experience other untoward and unwelcome events in our lives, we suffer. We suffer as whole persons: body, mind, and spirit bear the burden of the disease, accident, or other violation of the integrity we assign to ourselves, that sense we have of being a real person—a whole person—in a real world. We know who we are when we put our hands on our bodies in the bath, get dressed, or are touched by another. We know ourselves as individuals, as unique persons with a past that defines so much of who we are now. We live in the present, creating each day the self we are becoming;

but we also think about the future, near and distant, that will tell us and the world what we have become. When we, or those close to us, become sick or disabled, what we assumed was a whole person is radically altered; the present becomes a time of trial and the future suddenly and frighteningly becomes questionable, foreshortened.

A shocking part of the experience of being sick is the acute and unexpected focus on the body as our source of suffering, so often expressed as a sense of betrayal by an intimate friend from whom we never expected failure. We put our hands on our bodies in the middle of the night; is this really happening? Although we live our lives in our bodies, we spend little time with such a sharp concentration on them. We shower and shave, we put on our makeup with care, and we perform other bodily tasks without a lot of fixation on the functions themselves. So much taken for granted! With sickness, all this changes, and our bodies are center stage. The importance of understanding bodily suffering is central to the practice of medicine, underlying so much of current and ongoing concerns for the care of seriously ill and dying persons. Major worries of the public and of the professions these days center on the treatment of persons who are dying, who are fearful of inadequate care and abandonment, and who do not know what is to be done. In this chapter I will discuss the suffering we know in our bodies, and the influences suffering has on us as we live our lives. Bodily suffering is a nightmare we would avoid if at all possible. The suffering in mind and spirit that we will know will be considered in subsequent chapters.

Living in a Body

We live our lives in our bodies. Whether we are a newborn baby or an "ancient of days," we are in a physical body. Whether a professional athlete at the peak of a career, a paralyzed person living in a wheelchair, a child with a recent liver transplant, or a prostitute on the street, we live out this life in this body. What happens to this body is a major determinant of who we are: how we live, the loyalties we hold, the ultimate choices we make for ourselves and for others.

There are innumerable wonders to this bodily existence, and we know them in each moment. Our hearts beat and we breathe almost imperceptibly, rarely knowing that these crucial functions go on without our help. We see, we hear, we touch and feel, we smell, and we taste; or at least, most of us do, or have. One of the central surprises in life that we may translate into suffering is the loss of our sensibilities—the five contacts we make with our world. The surprise of loss comes because it is so unexpected. The ultimate loss is our dying to this world, the death of this body.

When we become ill we awaken to our bodies. Forgotten had been the richness of our senses, the significance of our work, the joys of the simplest physical acts done with intention. Always expected to be there at our service, suddenly the reliability of the body is brought into question. Our attention shifts to the functions of our body: the simplest of tasks can become a major hurdle requiring concentration and an inordinate amount of time to accomplish. Tying shoelaces, brushing teeth, and getting out of bed become chores that may not be carried off. Where before we assumed, of course, that the body would do what we wanted it to do, now we must attend to the details, careful to avoid situations where we will falter and hurt ourselves or appear foolish before strangers. We "tune in" to the body, as if listening for the slightest knock in the engine, the squeak that will need oil, the faintest suggestion that something is going wrong, an impending breakdown of the entire system. For persons who are being treated for serious diseases and are currently well and in remission or assumed cured, this constant monitoring of the body is like sitting on a time bomb, waiting for that earliest clue that the dreaded disease is reappearing. When we are well, the future seems almost without limit; in fact, we think of the future in terms of what we will do, get, or be. When we are unsure of the future because of a disease that threatens life itself, the future becomes truncated and questionable.

We presume that we will always be able to hear the organist play "Sheep May Safely Graze," watch the sun set and rise, smell the newly cut grass, hold the hand of the child, go to the movies, taste the delightful subtle differences between Italian and French roast espresso coffees. These senses are so ordinary, so common and expected in daily life, that their loss is inconceivable until we know it. This importance of this way of knowing ourselves, this acute awareness of the world around us in all its everyday wonder, awe, and simplicity, may only be recognized for the first time when we imagine the possibility of its loss. Over and over again we hear stories that recount the sadness of persons discovering that their goals and passions, their purposes and accomplishments turned to ashes in their hands when life itself was threatened. What defined them to others as to themselves is to simply disappear. The unanticipated possibility that life could end brings into exquisitely sharp question what we have assumed to be the cornerstones of our lives. A student translated her conversations with her patient-teacher into this talented fiction.

> When I first became ill—that is, when I first realized how seriously ill I was—I spent hours on my stomach on the carpet, nose to nose with my cat. "You have no idea how good you have it," I explained to him. The funny thing is that I will probably outlive him; he is in the twilight of his years, not counting his reincarnations, if you believe that sort of thing, which I don't, at least not anymore. There isn't much I haven't tried in the way of religions these last months. I'm floundering for a framework, a packing crate for this burden, this knowledge that I am dying and that this consciousness that simply *is* won't *be* anymore.[1]

A cause of pervasive agony is the thought that we will die never having really lived in ways that would show us as whole persons, responsible, affectionate, and a contributor to our culture. Suffering as regret is a sad ending to a life. I will discuss several categories of suffering tied to our understanding of ourselves as bodies that have reached a new, and distressingly unexpected, crossroad.

Suffering as Loss

She was a friend, the mother of children I had cared for in my practice. She was hospitalized now, and dying. She said,

You have to get used to it. Some things one has to give up, just plain will never happen again. I'm very fond of English marmalade—I make it in January; I'll never make that again because it is too tiring. . . . It is disheartening—the future brings with it nothing but death.

Experience has taught me that the touch of the hand, holding hands, can be the most comforting and intimate thing in the world. Holding the hand—that last ten seconds, gives the patient something that he can carry with him . . . thinking about the fact that he will never eat a peanut butter sandwich again.[2]

The symbolism of the marmalade and the sandwich are powerful reminders of the impact on us, the suffering we will endure, with that final deprivation of the simplest things we do: eat, talk, hold hands, be with friends. There is also the sad knowledge that we shall lose the touch of the hand of other persons, such a poignant reminder of the powerful simplicity of our common existence, a pensive question to caregivers about the innate significance of taking the hand of another in ours as comfort.

We suffer when we lose what is important to us. The loss of nonessentials can be annoying, making us angry, frustrated, even sad. Sometimes, however, we can laugh about the importance we attached to things that, now gone, turned out to be quite peripheral to our lives. But this is rarely true of the loss of functions of our bodies. We are our bodies. We live in them, work with them, find our pleasures through them. When young we are proud of them: their attractiveness; their skills in sports, singing, dancing, threading a needle, playing a musical instrument, tying sailor knots. The years of our lives move on, and there are unwelcome hints that changes are subtly taking place. We slow down, have aches and pains, tire more quickly, need reading glasses and, perhaps, a hearing aid, and have occasional sicknesses that annoy us. These are intimations of what lies ahead for all of us. All of these bothersome, seemingly trivial annoyances become glaringly apparent with serious disease.

Again, it is loss that causes our suffering. These are losses that we project into the future. We realize, with surprise, that the losses will accumulate, not diminish. We will become more dependent upon others, and our confidence in being in control of our lives is shaken. What we know as autonomy, the right to make the laws that govern our inner lives and determine our values, declines with sickness. For us, our nurturance, education and training, political experiences, and personal relationships are built upon a deeply ingrained sense of personal liberty and freedom to do, to be, and to become. We are seriously disturbed when illness causes a retreat from positions we cherish. With progression of disease, there is progressive loss of our self-control. For many of us this loss of self-control symbolizes all the other losses of sickness; we realize that things will not get better, just worse.

We are sensitive to this loss of independence; it is a prominent cause of our suffering. The frustration associated with increasing reliance on others for the tasks of everyday living can cause depression, adding to the problems we already have. Many of us associate loss of independence with loss of our very personhood. "I'd rather do it myself" is a common comment, even by those for whom the work in question, of no great import, will nevertheless consume a lot of time. We do not like to build a large store of indebtedness to others for the help they give us. In a very basic way we suffer when we realize we will not be able to repay the time and effort that others have expended in our care. We forget that we, in caring for our children and then our parents, in the professional lives we live, in the service organizations we support, and our quick responses to the needs of friends and strangers, are giving of ourselves, and usually without expectation of reward. We see these duties and services rather as expressions of our being persons in community, part of a chain of humanity.

We suffer when the pleasures we know and learned to treasure are taken away by our physical inability to enjoy them anymore. When we no longer can read, work in the garden, repair a damaged appliance, hold a grandchild, go to the Little League baseball game, balance the checkbook, or drive the car—we suffer because we are losing some of the definers of our lives. This is, of course, yet another area of our lives where support and encouragement, education and evaluation of personal goals are essential in the care of seriously ill patients. The roles of caregivers of the seriously ill will be developed later, and the central position of the patient as teacher will be discussed fully.

For many of us, our bodies are a primary avenue of expression of who we are and what we do. Certainly, our sexuality is detailed in our physical responses and encounters with the one we love. But reproduction of the species is not the only purpose of sexual intercourse. Human beings are unique in seeking and showing powerful expressions of their love in their sexuality. We are the only animal species that makes love face to face, a remarkable symbol of the centrality of choice in our loving. We reveal an intimate aspect of our whole person; we expose ourselves, in various ways, to another in most vulnerable ways. Certainly, loss of this function, so deeply ingrained in us since prehistoric times, is a cause of our suffering. Recognition of the significance of this loss opens the possibility of healing, if not curing, some of that loss by sensitive attention of health professionals.

Failure to grasp the enduring importance of our bodies to our understanding of who we are in this world can be painful and damaging to patients who have lost control of a significant part of the body. The sorrow we see in the tragedy of loss is shown in this encounter that I watched on ward rounds.

The young man was hospitalized after an automobile accident that left him paralyzed from the waist down. He lay in the bed, staring out the window at the fall afternoon, the type of day when he would be playing football for his college. In the earliest stages of his treatments, he had little understanding of what had happened to him, and of what the future held for him; he was only now beginning to realize the magnitude of his predicament. The bleakness of his future had not yet been fully described. The orthopedic resident, a woman, stopped by on morning rounds and asked him how he was feeling. She continued her conversation by asking him what he liked to do, what he was good at, what part of college was most challenging to him. He responded quickly and enthusiastically with an enlivened description of his long interest in athletics; he told of his pleasure and sense of accomplishment at playing the major sport of each season—football, basketball, and baseball; he was a bit embarrassed when he mentioned his awards. There was a moment of silence. The doctor looked him in the eye, and without any expression on her face, told him he had better learn to enjoy reading since he would never walk again. She turned away from his bedside and left the room.

How does one describe the desolation so painfully chiseled in the face of the young man, or the anger others felt toward the heartless physician? Suffering was never more clearly evident than at that moment.

What was so visible in the despair of that young man at that time of terror was his aloneness in his world. He could not even imagine what it meant to be unable to move. His physical disability separated him, at least at that moment, from the rest of us. We could not fully understand his torment, although we would say that we were in sympathy with him. Stricken by fate to lose what seemed most precious to him, he was alone in the universe. We realized that we never fully grasp the meaning of loss until we know it ourselves. No words of reassurance, no comfort of embrace, no preaching about hope would be of avail in relieving the frightening sense of utter loneliness this man knew to the very depths of his being. The work required to make amends for the inhumane behavior of the doctor and to relieve the suffering brought about by the loss of the body he knew and treasured will require an intensity of effort and a degree of tenderness by others that will declare their professional and personal characteristics to the world.

As is so clearly shown by the story of the young athlete, sickness limits choice. For many of us, choosing this rather than that, going here rather than there, being this person rather than that person are basic decisions that tell us and others who we are. The work we do, the roles we play in society, the burdens and responsibilities we assume, and the joys and pleasures we seek are ours to choose. We do not imagine ourselves otherwise until we are forced to a standstill by disease. With sickness, our defining characteristics become limited in a gradually narrowing circle as the focus becomes more and more the day-by-day living with disease. Choice is a defining sign of a free life in a society whose restraints are only those that keep us from invading the private lives of others. We do what we wish to do as long as we do not inflict limits on the freedom of others to do the same. It is obvious in our society that choice is closely bound to social and financial status, race, and freedom of opportunities for education and work. With sickness comes an ever sharper narrowing of freedom. We are now held within the obvious boundaries imposed by physical and psychological disability, the needs we have for assistance from others, and the anxiety we soon know as we project ourselves into the future. Choice, this assumed freedom to become what we can and do what we would, is an early casualty of sickness. To our dismay we are diminished as persons, becoming less than we were, and far less than we hoped we could be.

Pain and Suffering

Pain, in its many and varied forms, is a major cause of suffering. We all know pain as a part of the human experience. The thumb is hit with the hammer; a baby is delivered; a kidney stone is passed; the cancer has spread to the spine; a coronary artery is suddenly blocked by a small sclerotic fragment: all these cause pain, but we interpret them quite differently. Much of our pain is passing, a source of irritation and annoyance, often a cause for distress and anxiety, but not of suffering. A characteristic of the pain we associate with suffering, the kind that is experienced with serious illness or accident, is a peculiar sense of loss of real time: past, present, and future seem to blend together into a continuum as the inner time of the pain cancels our outer, or clock, time. The experience of a friend is illustrative.

He was in the hospital with a high fever, pneumonia, and severe back pain whose cause was unknown and treatment not clear. Throughout the day he lost track of time as he focused on his pain that would not let up. He tried to read, he watched some television without much understanding, but the pain was right there in front of him, his unwanted companion. He was convinced that it must be at least midafternoon by now, and was distressed to learn that it was barely midmorning. His

usual accurate estimate of the time of the day was lost in the dim room;
his pain completely distorted the reality of each moment.

S. Kay Toombs writes in *The Learning of Illness,*

> the patient experiences his or her illness in its immediacy in terms
> of the ongoing flow of "lived" time. If one is in pain, for example,
> each flicker of pain does not represent a discrete, atomic instant
> along a time-line, but rather a continuum of discomfort in which
> past and future pains coalesce into a stagnating present. . . . In the
> preoccupation with the here and now, the person who is ill pays
> little attention to clock time. Minutes may seem like hours, hours
> like days.[3]

Pain becomes a source of suffering when we realize its cause and
significance for our lives are deemed serious. The first function of our
thought is usually to learn the cause of the pain, to hear the diagnosis.
Put simply, if it is the hammer hitting the thumb, its significance is
minimal. If the bone pain is due to the unexpected and unbelievable
diagnosis of metastatic cancer, both the present diagnosis, possible
treatments, and the projection into the future are ominous. There
are, therefore, two varieties of suffering: the first is that associated
with the immediate pain and treatment; the second is the long-range
outlook, the reflection on what this diagnosis signifies for the future
in terms of pain, loss of independence, and the possibility of death.
Here pain assumes center stage and becomes a primary cause for suffering, both immediate and potential. For the patient, the specter of
unremitting pain, stretching endlessly into the future, becomes a terrifying reality, profoundly debilitating, and a source of suffering.

Our personal concerns about our pain appear as questions. What
is the cause of the pain? What does the pain mean? If there is a ready
explanation, pain is usually easier to manage. Even though the diagnosis is serious, the outlook unclear, and the possibilities for successful therapy dubious, many persons report less suffering than when
all the questions are up in the air, opinions are contradictory, and
options vague. Even with the pain, suffering seems less when all inter-

ested parties know what is going on, what steps need to be taken, what the statistics show. When caregivers are unsure about the clinical aspects of the case—diagnosis, treatment, and prognosis—the anxiety and the suffering of the patient are certain to be accentuated. Eric J. Cassell writes in *The Nature of Suffering*,

> [P]eople in pain frequently report suffering from pain when they feel out of control, when the pain is overwhelming, when the source of the pain is unknown, when the meaning of the pain is dire, or when the pain is apparently without end.
>
> In these situations, persons perceive pain as a threat to their continued existence—not merely to their lives but their integrity as persons. That this is the relation of pain to suffering is strongly suggested by the fact that suffering can often be relieved *in the presence of continued pain,* by making the source of the pain known, changing its meaning, and demonstrating that it can be controlled and that an end is in sight.[4]

The Significance of Suffering

All that I have noted suggests that suffering has no positive aspects at all for us. Certainly, as patients, the *presence* of suffering in our life is not a welcome one. It is, however, a part of life and a part that can enrich, humble, and inform us of the vagaries of this human existence. For us as caregivers, understanding as best we can what suffering entails encourages and supports a developed and studied compassion and a defining willingness to be with and for others. Wherever we are on our personal journey, we can learn of ourselves by watching the experiences of others, committing ourselves to their welfare, and accepting responsibility for those close to us. Suffering awakens us to our bodies, shifting attention from outside interests to that center of our being, our bodies. We are bodies in all those ways I discussed. Accepting the transience of life as definitive of the existence of all that lives can help us do the work of caring.

The suffering that we see and know is, as suggested above, a result of the inevitable conquest of our bodies by a disease process that destroys them. We lose the integrity of the self, that precious commodity we admire in others as we cherish it in ourselves. As Toombs writes,

> Illness is primarily experienced as a fundamental *loss of wholeness*. . . .
> [T]his loss of wholeness manifests itself in the awareness of bodily disruption or impairment an awareness that is not so much a simple recognition of specific symptoms . . . as it is a profound sense of the loss of total bodily integrity. The body can no longer be taken for granted or ignored. It has seemingly assumed an opposing "will" of its own, beyond the control of the self. Rather than functioning effectively at the bidding of the self, the body-in-pain or the body-malfunctioning thwarts plans, impedes choices, renders actions impossible.[5]

There is a recognition that what has happened—the disease—is beyond comprehension either biologically or philosophically. For many of us, it is sickness that brings us abruptly to the realization that life is tenuous, that we all live on borrowed time.

But there are other ways in which we manifest integrity and live out a life in the face of disease and hardship and threat. We do have other parts to ourselves, divisions that I broadly label as our mind and our spirit. These, as well as the body, will know suffering when sickness becomes our bedfellow. How we suffer in these areas will be discussed in succeeding chapters. The function of this study is to show the nature of sufferings that we know, learn from patients what constitutes human suffering, and learn also how we can help alleviate suffering. After all, who better than sick persons can teach us the fundamentals of compassionate care and the relief of human suffering.

Notes

1. E. Choo, personal communication, 1996.
2. C. Barnard, recorded interview, 1979.
3. S. Kay Toombs, *The Meaning of Illness* (Dordrecht: Kluwer Academic Publishers, 1992), 15.

4. Eric J. Cassell, *The Nature of Suffering* (New York: Oxford University Press, 1991), 36.

5. Toombs, *The Meaning of Illness,* 90.

6

"In a Situation That Involves the End"

My wife said, "I wouldn't have missed these last two months for anything; they are the best two months of my life." In many ways it was
about as wonderful a conclusion as one could expect. I learned a
great deal about what love is. . . . I think, in a situation that involves
the end, everything becomes more powerful, more important, more
emphatic, including love. And it could be said that [she], in those
last few months, learned to love in a new and deeper way than she
knew before; something new, something deeper, something finer;
and in a way it made the whole experience worthwhile.[1]

This comment on one specific aspect of the last months of his
wife's life is poignant, powerful, and discouraging; there is a sadness in it. The reader senses a hint of regret that this realization of a
deeper meaning of love for her came so late. But there is hope also in
knowing that we can always learn more about the meanings of our
relationships with others. This brief vignette is a common theme in
human experience when we truly understand that the end is
approaching and we shall no longer have seemingly unlimited time to
enjoy this life. There is, after all, a continuity in our experiences of

living that is paralleled in our experiences of dying. Life and death are a continuum.

Utterly unrealistic though we know it to be, many of us act as if life went on forever. As we pursue our often humdrum and repetitious lives we are forever planning for tomorrow, letting this day slip by as we ignore the possibilities for deepening our relationships with others and enriching the social and intellectual lives we say we cherish. A most difficult task is to live each day to its fullness in the way we live it out. It is so inconceivable that it might be the beginning of our ending. And yet, in our minds we surely know this as a possibility, unwelcome though it is. The diagnosis of a serious, perhaps life-threatening disease brings an instant halt to long-term planning and precipitates a number of emotional responses that cause suffering, sadness, and misery. Understanding these feelings and their impact upon us are important tasks for both the persons who are sick and for those caring for them, be they professional healthcare providers or family and friends. As persons we can suffer as much in our emotions and our feelings as we can in our bodies, perhaps even more. An immediate example suggested to us by the anecdote above is that of regret: there is suddenly no time for enhancing a segment of the inner self that now has become so worthwhile.

An Avalanche of Feelings

With confirmation of the diagnosis of a menacing disease can come an outpouring of emotions, usually strong and clear. These emotions are very often negative in content, destructive of our responses and relationships. There can be such wild fancies about the as yet unknown and terrifying significance of this disease for this person. Our impressive human imagination is such a powerful actor in our lives, both in our inner lives lived out in our minds, and also in our outer lives as creative persons in the arts, sciences, politics, domestic joys and pleasures, and everyday tasks at work or in the garden. With imagination we visualize possibilities and utopias—heavens and hells—and conjure up relationships that will enrich and beautify our world and show us forth as realized human beings who, with honesty, compassion, and vigilance did the work that needed to be done. With the diagnosis of serious disease and its placing a halter on those hopes, we finally understand that all does come to an end, something we knew but which we did not allow to interpret our lives. Now, with the reality of an ending, we suffer with the loss of that desired future. Sigmund Freud thought that it was impossible for us to imagine ourselves as dead, that death was an actuality, a conception that we could not truly grasp. I do not agree with this, but it is impossible to prove one way or the other. It is difficult to comprehend not being here in this world that I see about me. But it is a reality that we must encounter, and encounter it without guilt over the person we did not become or the things we did not do.

A major emotion we know in many aspects of our lives is anxiety. To be anxious is to be unsure of what the future holds for us: what can happen, and when? There are a number of possibilities, particularly in our inventive minds, but it is unclear what the odds are for this one or for that. Neither we nor anyone else knows or will tell us what to expect at this time. "Why am I so tired and losing weight? I seem so pale; what does that mean? I do not understand those vague medical words, and the doctor seems to be avoiding telling me what is the matter. I am terrified, but I don't know of what!" We are afraid to ask those frightening questions, afraid that our worst fears will become actualities. Anxiety is a most unwelcome visitor since there is little that we or another can do to relieve it. To be anxious is to suffer, and the drain on the emotions is severe because it is so difficult to turn anxiety aside. A defining characteristic of anxiety is the failure of reassurance—in the absence of proof—to free us from its miserable effects.

Fear, on the other hand, is a response to a life-threatening disease that is rational because it is a response to reality. It is an emotional form of suffering that can be understood, confronted, and frequently resolved by varied caregivers: physicians, nurses, social workers, clergy, and family. There are very real fears when we become sick, especially if the disease is possibly fatal. This is the time when we begin to suffer in ways that are more devastating than the physical ones. An entire gamut of emotions descends upon us as all the parts of our lives—interior, familial, social, political, professional—suddenly are threatened. What lies ahead? We, being defined so much by these personal aspects of ourselves, can be overwhelmed by our awareness that they will disappear when we die. These are real fears, certainly matching the fears we have about pain, embarrassing loss of bodily and mental functions, undesirable forms of treatment, and the possibility of being alone at the end. Another source of fear is the burden that sickness brings on others; financial as well as personal questions are paramount for many persons when the finality of the outcome is apparent. The cost of care in the draining of resources essential to our children and our grandchildren causes suffering since the sick person is often powerless to alter the course of events. Our emotional resources are also depleted by the erosion of self and others by severe illness. These are fears that are fully understandable. The fact that separates fear from anxiety is that fear is directed at specific targets and does not have the vagueness and the unanswerable nature of anxiety. The objects of fear can be confronted and managed, relieving the patient of much of the emotional suffering we anticipate when serious illness envelopes our lives. It is the suffering caused by fear that can be managed and relieved, as anxiety cannot be. This relief of fear is a major duty of caregivers.

A Sense of Regret

In this deluge of emotions upon us when we are seriously ill, there are several negative ones we must be clear about since caregivers should be sensitive in recognizing them and their significance for healing and caring. These are feelings that we have when things go badly for us, emotional responses to the reality of the situation that can be understood as real and appropriate by others and then addressed as actual parts of the illness. Regret is just such a feeling. When the future is foreshortened, when detachment from persons, places, pleasures, and treasures is suddenly a distinct possibility, if not a reality, we have regrets. These feelings are powerful causes of suffering because they have a "might-have-been" quality that haunts us. We suffer when we know that accepted parts of our lives will be severed: relationships with children, parents, and friends will end; creative work that has engaged us for decades will be done no more; the sources of our pleasures—art and music, nature, sexuality, learning, teaching—will be no more. These losses are commonly associated with regret, with that feeling that we might have done otherwise, spoken differently, been more attentive to what now seems so obvious, walked that extra mile with the needy stranger. Regret is a strong negative force upon us when we feel threatened by loss of our very being. A secondary effect of this regret is often anger directed within, disgust with the missed opportunities to be with and for others for whom we care, and a sense of shame for those things done and left undone by us. Very few of us become the person we hoped to be. This self-abasement is a source of suffering when regrets about our unchangeable past become part of our sickness.

A Different Person Now

We suffer when we see the alterations caused by disease in the self we knew in the past. We may become physically disabled, even deformed, seemingly unworthy of the love of those who loved us before. We may well loathe what we have become, suffering in dread of rejection by others we value. When we are no longer like others in appearance, in physical capabilities, and in the roles we played, we fear that we shall be cast out of our circle of family and friends, shunned by the very ones we counted on for support, persons we have supported in the past. For some persons this is a reality. Certain diseases carry a strong negative connotation, inducing fear of contagion, anxiety about caring for the sick one, and often the suggestion that the disease is evil.

She was a nun and a teacher in the medical-school course who was recently diagnosed with metastatic breast cancer. A teacher for many years, she lived in a community of her order. One of her sad surprises when her diagnosis became known was the sudden and unexpected shift in her relationships. Some nuns in her order to whom she had been a close friend abandoned her, became distant and disinterested in her progress. She felt untouchable, separated from trusted colleagues. To her amazement, other nuns who had been only acquaintances became friends in helping care for her, taking on her tasks, assuring her comfort and rest. For the patient this was a revelation, helping her accept the different person that the disease had made of her, assuring her of support, and speaking to the kindnesses of others when suffering is real and palpable. What had happened to her body was not of her doing, and others recognized this and accepted her as she was and would become. The rejection by her former friends was painful but she understood their anxieties and forgave them.

I have heard about these responses from a number of patients. Occasionally, even family members will retreat from the sick person, a very distressing reaction to sickness. But then, someone in the neighborhood hears about the sick person, knocks on the door, asking if they can help in driving to the clinic, shopping, taking the children to school. The sense of relief, the confirmation of community, and the warmth of new friendships can be very supportive when anxiety is nearly overwhelming.

An interesting reversal in roles can occur in some families when the patient assumes responsibility for the emotional support of others who are devastated by what will happen to *them* when mother, father, wife, or child dies. Patients often must continue their previous roles as organizer, definer, comforter, and educator of others despite the obvious alteration in their physical state. It is not unusual for children who are dying to feel very protective of their parents and support them in their denial of what is occurring.

Another source of emotional suffering is the shame we know when our bodies disappoint us in their ordinary functions. There are many distressing symptoms during the last months of dying: difficulty in breathing, nausea and vomiting, insomnia and mental confusion, and fatigue. Loss of control of bowel and bladder is a marked source of self-disgust and suffering. To need to be cared for like a diapered baby, to be afraid to go out of the house for fear of an intimate accident, and to be unable to care for oneself are sources of profound embarrassment and frustration. We can easily abhor ourselves when the simplest of private tasks can no longer be done by us. In our suffering, we feel betrayed by our bodies, outcasts from the regular order of society. It is difficult indeed to be at ease and comfortable in these circumstances; we can be taught how to alleviate at least some of the suffering.

Another response that some of us make to the anxieties and the fears that we know when we get sick is profoundly negative in its effects. One of the patients in the medical-school course was a most informative and revealing teacher for the students. A young woman who had worked in the entertainment world and knew many celebrities in her social life, she received a bone-marrow transplant that failed to take. Her prognosis was poor and she was obviously in pain and sad. But she also took on an exceedingly negative approach to herself and to her world. Everyone else was to blame for her miseries: doctors, nurses, friends, and colleagues; all had, in some way, contributed to her present distressing state. Her language was foul, her comments cutting and hurtful to those attempting to care for her, and she had effectively isolated herself from all who could possibly be of help. The medical students were able to learn from her the terrors associated with removal of the self from others, and the occasional person who remains completely alone and cannot be reached. Although it is so difficult to do, we must learn to move toward, rather than away from, such persons, hoping to overcome their powerful feeling of self-rejection.

Whose Fault Is This?

Guilt is a feeling we all know well that causes profound suffering; since the relief of suffering is a declared goal and commitment of those who care for the sick, understanding the impact of guilt on us is essential. There are many sources of our feelings of guilt, and I shall discuss a few of them.

1. When we realize that we are sick with a disease that may cause our death, we are brought into sharp confrontation with ourselves, all

of ourselves. We review our lives to analyze our goals in this life: were they really what we wanted, were they worth the life we dedicated to them? Henry David Thoreau was concerned with these questions, so wisely discussed in his book *Walden*.

> I went to the woods because I wished to live deliberately, to front only the essential facts of life, and see if I could not learn what it had to teach, and not, when I came to die, discover that I had not lived. I did not wish to live what was not life, living is so dear; . . . .[2]

Roger C. Bone, a prominent physician and a professor of medicine, dying with metastatic renal cancer writes,

> It would be untruthful to say I look forward to dying. I would rather live another 20 or 30 years, grow old with my wife, watch my two daughters mature, play with my grandchildren, and continue to deepen my appreciation for good literature, for great music, and, above all else, for nature. This is not, on balance, a great deal to ask for, and yet it is everything. . . . If I were granted 20 more years, I would certainly continue my research, but with one difference: it would not be the controlling factor in my life. One of the things I have learned from the process of my dying is that the most important things in the process of my living were not what I—and most others—usually think are important. They are rather in the category of things we usually take for granted—health, family, friends, and a relationship with our Creator.[3]

Were the goals we set, the promises we made, and the hopes we entertained the ones we now continue to support and affirm? Those who care for the sick must be alert to these questions—often asked obliquely—so that the feelings of guilt that patients have can be clearly distinguished, discussed, and opportunities for redefining priorities and purposes restated and lived in the remaining time. This confrontation with the self suddenly and unexpectedly presented by illness can be an enlightening and freeing experience assisted by those of us aware of underlying concerns, and helpful in their definition and discussion.

2. What role do we play in the causation of our disease? There is no question that personal behavior can be the primary cause of diseases that are fatal. We know of so many now: smoking cigarettes is both a primary cause of lung cancer and a contributing factor in many other diseases that cause death. These have been very well documented in medical research and are known by the public. Diet is also a prominent factor in diseases that are life-threatening. Obesity, a diet high in fat and cholesterol, excessive alcohol use, and many other habitual acts are factors causing diseases that kill. Personal habits and behavior cause accidents that maim and kill, acts for which personal responsibility must be recognized, a persistent source of guilt for the suffering we have brought on ourselves and on others by behavior that could have been avoided. Herein lies the sadness of bad decisions and actions: we hurt others in many ways, and there is no making up for that hurt, no removing that suffering. Our guilt is firmly established. When bad things happen to us are we merely getting what we deserve, a certain retribution for errors, faults—even bad thoughts—for which we now are to pay the price?

3. The distinct possibility of death causes guilt when we realize that we will not accomplish what we had set out to do with our lives. Suddenly the future is closed off. We are known to ourselves and to others so often by work, by position in society and profession, and by reputation. Suddenly these are of no account as one faces the certainty of extinction. The functions of the body, the creations of the mind, the commitments of the heart and the soul are to be lost and barely remembered. What so defined us before is no longer relevant. A certain conviction of our integrity, our oneness or wholeness as a person in this world, is lost and our feelings of guilt can feel overwhelming.

4. Guilt is also caused by our realization of the effects that our sickness and dying will have on so many others: family and friends, colleagues and dependents, private and public roles that we accepted. The very relationships that defined a significant part of us are to be dissolved and abandoned by us. Not only are we to be alone in our misery, but we are bringing this upon others, made worse for many of us by the realization that we may have had a major role in the cause of the losses by our own neglect and ignorance.

Separated and Silent

A response to these feelings of guilt that we often assume when we assess our lives, the role we may have played in our imagined downfall, and the prospect of that life ending without our realizing our potentials is further suffering by isolating ourselves from others. Caregivers must be cautious because fear of abandonment is very strong in persons who are approaching their death. Over and over I have heard persons discuss, quite candidly, their expected and awaited death. For many of us, death as the end of life is an acknowledged fact that we would never deny. Our experiences as persons in this world make death a known, if undesirable, companion of the living. It is the act of dying that is a source of deep concern, even frightful and paralyzing anxiety for many. The central fear is that one would die alone, abandoned and without careful attention as life ebbed away.

Certainly central to the ongoing discussion and debate about how we die is this concern about being abandoned during our dying. There is, appropriately, very serious argument about the role of physicians in assisting their patients in dying, and about the dangers and fears of improper uses of assisted suicide in our culture. Again, the fears of the patients come together in this common concern over abandonment. This is not only an obvious anxiety about dying alone in a room separated from the rest of the hospital floor. It is also the very real possibility of dying without having one's wishes and plans accepted as legitimate by those caring for the patient or by the family responsible for deciding the course to be followed to the end.

Depression is a symptom and sign common when death becomes a distinct possibility. John Hinton, emeritus professor of psychiatry at the University of London, writes,

> When an individual is very ill and weak it can be difficult to distinguish exhaustion and physical discomfort from a troubled state of mind. . . . The signs and symptoms of depression and anxiety states are essentially those characteristic of these mood states whatever their source but likely to contain the particular fears and sorrows of dying. . . . Depression can range from a little quiet sadness, perhaps

tears, to unhappiness and social withdrawal. . . . It is not uncommon for onlookers to misinterpret the psychological changes.[4]

Professional caregivers, family members, and friends must be alert to this often hidden response to threatening disease. We must also be aware that depression is a condition treatable by both psychological and pharmacological means. A common error is found in the statement "I'd be depressed, too, if I had that disease," the improper assumption being that nothing can be done about it.

Another source of silent suffering is occasioned by the silence of those close to the patient about what is happening. An old tradition holds to withholding the seriousness of the medical condition and proposed treatments from the patient, only revealing this information to responsible relatives. This scenario, common everywhere until a few decades ago, was altered radically in the United States with the development of the profession of biomedical ethics. Both academic and governmental policies were put into place that assured patients that their informed consent would be needed before anything was done to them, that information would be held in confidence, and, for our purposes, the patient would know the facts of the diagnosis and the prognosis. Only in this way could intelligent and informed decisions be made by the patient about treatment plans. Many other countries still do not follow this type of guideline; patients may appear to know little about their medical and surgical problems. Of course, a common finding is that the patient does know, from all that has been done and the attitudes of caregivers and family, that all is not well. There is often a conspiracy of silence so that no one speaks to what all know.

This situation, where neither patient nor family speaks to the obvious issues, can cause sadness and suffering for all parties. A medical student reports on one of his interviews with his patient, an older man hospitalized for chemotherapy.

It was midmorning, and the patient was describing in detail the onset of his disease, the medical attention he sought and received, and his disturbing personal inner responses to the frightening experience. The medical student was silent and fully absorbed in the gripping story he was

hearing, a soul-searching account of a startling encounter with the pos-
sibility of becoming very sick and possibly dying in the near future. As
the patient talked, and the student listened, almost hypnotized by the
words, the door to the room opened and the patient's wife appeared,
smiling and cheerful. Without a second's pause or change in facial or
vocal expression, the patient broke off in midsentence his description of
the effects of chemotherapy and began to describe his grandchildren. His
wife took off her jacket, said hello to them, and said she was off to get a
cup of coffee and would be right back. As she left the room, the patient,
again without any alteration in speech or appearance, returned
promptly to his previous account of his progress with his cancer.

The medical student was silent as he reflected on the sadness this man
must feel facing his trials essentially alone. When his wife returned,
current baseball scores were the new and immediate topic. The implications of this vignette are serious for all concerned and of prime
importance for caregivers and for families when serious disease must
be lived with and its meanings confronted.

A corollary to this experience of minimal communication between patient and family is the unfortunately all-too-common lack of
effective and accurate communication between physician and patient.

The patient, Steve, was newly diagnosed with leukemia. As he lay in his
hospital bed he could hear the staff coming down the hall making their
morning rounds. They stood outside his closed door, and he could hear
them talk, although indistinctly. Steve heard one of the doctors say the
word "cancer," followed by laughter. The door opened, the staff came in,
asked him how he was without calling him by name, and left in a few
minutes, giving him no information about his disease and the possibili-
ties and options for treatment. Steve was distressed and angry as he told
me of this encounter. Sadly, his response was self-defeating. He said, "If
they aren't going to tell me anything, I'm not going to tell them any-
thing!" He later told me of his experience at his first appointment in the
medical oncology clinic. The doctor said that chemotherapy was the
treatment of choice. Steve asked what chemotherapy is; the doctor replied,
"It'll either cure you or kill you." Steve and his wife burst into tears and

left; it was weeks before they could be convinced to return to the clinic for his treatment.

The Functions of Forgiveness

As we have seen, when we become seriously ill and the possibility of death in the near future is a reality, many of us take a close look at our lives. We question our values, our commitments, and the places where we have invested our very selves. Who is important to me? What work do I do, and for what end? As did Dr. Bone, the physician noted above on page 92, we may, quite unexpectedly, realize that we must review and perhaps repeal some of the promises we made. Another aspect of this life review is a frequently painful acknowledgment that we need both to forgive and to be forgiven. One of the wake-up calls we receive when time is suddenly running short is the realization that there have been events and encounters, commitments and promises, assurances and duties that have been bypassed, ignored, and perhaps forgotten.

The closer the bonds we have with others, the more susceptible we can be to misunderstandings and to giving and receiving hurts and sorrows. Joy and happiness are not the only rewards for family life as parent or child, and most of us have been both. I am sure that many of us recall going to bed, promising ourselves that tomorrow we would be a good parent, only to have that promise shattered before breakfast was half over. We remember all too well the words we wish we had never spoken. Most of us have broken vows of one kind or another to others and to ourselves. All this adds up, when serious and life-threatening disease appears, to a heavy sense of regret and a very real suffering for what can never, it seems, be made right. The suffering we know when we see clearly what we have done and not done in our past is most real and painful. This suffering is often done in silence because we are embarrassed to talk about it, even with those closest to us, those often whom we have hurt and who have hurt us. Estrangement within families is common and a certain source of suffering, whether we are willing to admit to it or not.

She was old and fragile, dying of advanced cancer that was long past any possibility for treatment other than control of her pain. She was somber and withdrawn, hardly speaking to anyone, staff or family. The cancer progressed inexorably and it was a wonder that she did not die; she just lay in bed, staring out the window, rarely speaking except to ask for water. Most of her family had come to be with her, and all marveled at her intransigence in not dying. Finally, a sister arrived from the other coast, a sibling from whom she had been estranged for years over an incident involving a young man desirable to both women. Over time and distance there was no opportunity or apparent wish for reconciliation, yet both women were ill at ease and each felt responsible for their failed friendship with the other. With that false sense of pride known to many of us, neither would make a move to see or talk to the other, and the bitterness just sat there. When her sister arrived in the hospital room, the rest of the family left, and the two women held hands, talked for a few minutes, shed their tears in silence. The dying woman then smiled, turned her face gently to the window, and died. She had both forgiven and been forgiven, and was now free to let her life end, confident that healing had been accomplished where it had been thought impossible.

Comment

When we become seriously ill with a disease that may bring our life to its end, we expect that there will be physical suffering. Diagnostic procedures and surgical treatments, nausea and weakness, pain and loss of control of bodily functions that are so private—all these and others will be sources of agony and misery for us. We anticipate that there will be effective help from professional caregivers that will alleviate much of this suffering. But we are an amazingly complex entity, this reality we call a person. What may surprise many of us is the emotional suffering that we will know when we are very sick. I have outlined some of the sources of this type of suffering so that we, as patients and as physicians, nurses, social workers, and other professionals, will be alert to their existence. Only as we anticipate this type of suffering can we assist the sick and sad in our care, alert to signs of anguish and torment.

Emotional suffering that we know in our minds and hearts is more difficult to assess than physical pain, and therefore more difficult to manage effectively. However, this type of suffering is an integral part of our sicknesses and must be searched for as diligently as we would the sources of physical suffering and pain. We have enough evidence from the words of others and our own searched minds to confirm the centrality of feelings to our understanding of ourselves. Integrity, that sought-after quality of the well-lived life, must be valued in the patient as well as the doctor and others who care for the sick. The sense of wholeness that we are examining as we look at suffering includes awareness of the body as the bearer of all we are, the vehicle that transports the person each of us is. Our sure confidence of ourselves as one—as integrated—also must consider the power of our emotions to inform, to show forth, to damage and destroy, and to alter the person we would be. Recognizing suffering in the mind is as crucial to knowing the care needed as is knowing the senses of the body.

Part of the purpose of this study is to assist us in understanding the self, in recognizing the qualities and the characteristics of a person, one like ourselves, who will someday become sick, have an accident or other event that will bring life to its close. In the process of that acted-out drama some of us will be called upon to care for the dying. To do this effectively and humanely requires understanding the sufferings I have noted.

There remains another part of the person, the spirit, that we must look at as a suffering segment of the whole. Our lives are spiritual in a number of ways, and not all in the traditions we commonly label as religious. I shall look next at some of the ways we suffer in matters of the spirit.

Notes

1. R. Sewall, in *A Sense of the Ending*, a film by the Connecticut Humanities Council, 1982.

2. Henry David Thoreau, *Walden,* ed J. Lyndon Shanley (Princeton, N.J.: Princeton University Press, 1971), 90.

3. Roger C. Bone, "Maumee: My Walden Pond," *JAMA,* 276 (December 25, 1996): 24, 1931.

4. J. Hinton, "Coping with Terminal Illness," in *The Experience of Illness* (London: Tavistock Publications, 1984), 231–32.

7

The Spirit Within

The prophet Ezekiel writes that God spoke to him in these words: "'I will put my spirit within you and you shall live, and I will place you on your own soil; and then you shall know that I, the LORD, have spoken and will act,' says the LORD."[1]

Many of us attest to the existence of a third part to our personalities, an important and defining segment we call the spirit. Not easily described, we have, nevertheless, over the thousands of years of our history, borne witness to the certainty of a union with the universe not limited to our bodies and minds. Many persons in our long and tumultuous history report a sense of awe before the majestic wonder of our unbelievably complex universe: from the assurance of astronomers that new stars are being formed at this very moment in a space that is beyond our wildest imaginings to the study by physicists of particles of matter smaller than the electron. Although the legends and myths of the dawn of the universe differ and the characters that play the roles in the dramas are not the same, our human history returns again and again to a belief in a creator. Others of us find our spiritual lives fulfilled in our relationships with others, particularly the oppressed, the suffering—all those in need of comfort. Without a belief in a transcendent God a realized life can be known in companionship—the sharing of bread—with fellow sojourners on this earthly pilgrimage. Certainly, traditional religious beliefs are not a condition for deeply compassionate care of those who require assistance. Existential thought of this century has—with power and clarity—held forth the richness of a life devoted to being with and for the sick, the prisoner, the sorrowing, and the dying. The writings of Albert Camus speak to our call to join those who suffer and to rebel against the causes of needless suffering. That rebellion becomes the direct expression of a spiritual faith that, for some of us, is as meaningful as belief in God. Discovering and knowing the self become both the rewards and the driving forces for caring for others.

I think that we all have a god, a place of final confidence and trust, a vehicle through which we understand ourselves and what we know of this world. By no means must this god be found in any traditional religion or philosophy or psychology. But we each find that god, that foundation for living out our lives with some sense of purpose. Our god can be one of many options. Fame and fortune are the gods of many, as are the many and varied delights of the senses. We can put our confidence and our hope in intellect, in science, and in the creative arts. We can seek assurance in our control of the lives of others through politics, money, and sheer physical power. It is our option to choose the god who will be our ultimate source of reality and knowledge. We will use this god to justify and to describe the world we know. For we cannot explain the world, the physical and mental worlds that we inhabit. We can only describe what we think we see, be it a supernova or a chromosome. Why and for what purpose remain flights of imagined—often brilliantly imagined—fancy. There is no explanation for what we see and enjoy.

We use a language to describe our understandings and our experiences with creative activities, both of human and of divine origins. This language is ancient and yet holds its ground even today as we speak of spirit and of God. Throughout our history the word *spirit* is used to describe both the character of a creator and the part of us that responds in confidence and in hope to it. Spirit is also knowable in the significance of our relations with all other persons in this human adventure. In Western religious thought it is proposed that there is a spirit within us that responds to the Spirit that is understood as the way, the conduit, through which God is active in the world and thus knowable to us in varied guises. We speak to a concept of transcendence, a sense of knowing that there is a part of human experience that can get beyond the immediate, that "transcends," that is over and beyond ordinary daily life. The word *God* has been prominent in Western civilization as the name we ascribe to the creator and sustainer we confess to. Other cultures throughout our long history have living traditions that honor and worship gods as venerable and majestic, as profound and inspiring, as intimate and personal as the one I named. Again, a characteristic of our understanding of the nature of God and of our relationship to God is the quality of spirit that goes beyond any physical, emotional, or intellectual determinants. We commonly speak to our conviction that God is known as a Spirit by that part of us we call spirit. As with most of our lives, choices are constantly in process of being selected and lived through.

Since I was born, raised, and trained in the Christian tradition, I am limited to it in my understanding of what God and the life of the spirit mean. Even here, there are serious differences in how persons understand the spiritual component of life and the relationships we have with God. These differences have often been the source of the most destructive forces we can propel against those who believe otherwise, as our violent history testifies. We accept these differences as typical of the human enterprise; in fact they add to the diversity of faiths that we hold central to our lives. The addition of a spiritual component to human existence then adds the distinct possibility of suffering in matters of the spirit, not just the body and the mind. This suffering can be profound since it is often tied to the ways by which we understand our very being and our place in this world. Far beyond physical pain and suffering, and more intense than the sadness of failed personal relationships or fear and anxiety about the nature of our disease, is the awareness of meaninglessness that serious illness can bring upon us.

Loss of Meaning

For many persons, a loss of meaning for our lives is profoundly and deeply damaging, leaving one without confidence and without faith, bereft in a personal world abandoned by God. The experiences inherent in living with a life-threatening sickness raise questions known through the ages. Are we alone in this universe, sufferers from conditions that have no meaning, or is there a God who supports and cares? Is there any meaning to what happens to us as patients and as caregivers? How are we to understand the joys, the sorrows, the happiness and the sadness, the rewards and the sacrifices that all come to a close with our inevitable death and disappearance?

The central issue for our consideration of suffering that we know in our spiritual life is loss of meaning for that life. Disease brings on so suddenly the realization that life may very well end soon. John Donne (1571–1631), an English poet and Anglican priest, wrote witty and romantic poetry, satiric attacks on political figures of his day, and a series of reflections on his own very serious illness, probably typhus. Donne was remarkable in holding together in his writings the deep and abiding relationships between matter and spirit, body and soul. He sought with great care to understand the meanings of his religious faith for his life and his commitments. He noted that he had had three births: his natural one when he entered the world, his spiritual one when he was ordained into the ministry, and his supernatural one when he recovered from the disease that he expected would kill him. His meditations on that illness, called *Devotions Upon Emergent Occasions,* begin with this observation. I have taken the liberty to modernize his words.

> Variable, and therefore miserable condition of Man; this minute I was well, and am ill, this minute. I am surprised with a sudden change, and alteration to worse, and can impute it to no cause, nor call it by any name. We study *Health,* and we deliberate upon our *meats,* and *drink,* and *air,* and *exercises,* and we hew, and we polish every stone, that goes into that building; and so our *Health* is a long and regular work; but in a minute a cannon batters all, overthrows

all, demolishes all; a *sickness* unprevented for all our diligence, unsuspected for all our curiosity; nay, undeserved, if we consider only *disorder*, summons us, seizes us, possesses us, destroys us in an instant.[2]

For so many of us there is no explanation for our new and serious illness. We know that there are behavior patterns that are likely to cause fatal disease: smoking, hazardous chemicals in the workplace, diet, the ways in which we use alcohol and other drugs, and lifestyle patterns all have predictive value for serious diseases. Inheritance is certainly a factor in susceptibility to cancers, diabetes, cardiovascular accidents, and many other conditions. Inappropriate behavior and neglect of care for children and those dependent upon us can bring on their own catastrophes. But why now, at this time and in this place? What, if anything, can be the meaning of being stricken with serious disease? Is it a test of our faith or merely the working of impersonal fate? Is there specific meaning to suffering in the spirit, or is there no meaning to life other than what we actually live out in our few years? Does it all signify nothing other than just living, working, reproducing, and dying, hoping to have some enjoyment on the voyage? Are we abandoned to our fate: is what we see what there is?

The Search for Meaning

The busyness of our everyday life often precludes our search for the defining characteristics of that life. We are caught up in family matters, in the work that we do, and in the social and personal worlds that we live in. The unexpected appearance in our lives of serious disease quickly raises questions about the goals and the purposes of our daily living. What does my life mean? What foundation have I used upon which I have constructed my life? If I were to do this over again, would I choose the same means and ends? These are questions about the meaning of my life, central questions the answers to which tell you who I am. These are what I call spiritual questions, queries about the meaning of my life for me and for others, regardless of the foundations of our lives, the source of our confidence and functioning. I think that for many of us life is a search for a spirit that can be known, a sense of otherness in our lives that supports us and confirms us when there is obvious loss and failure. It is at times of sickness, when anxiety and loneliness can nearly overwhelm us, that being upheld in our suffering and pain is such a meaningful act. A very real form of suffering, as powerful as that of body and mind, can occur when our spiritual life is neglected.

One of the problems with the spiritual component of our lives is the inadequate preparation most of us have had in living out the spiritual journey needed for facing the ultimate questions that sickness so unexpectedly presents. Many of us have not pursued our education in matters of the spirit. We stopped going to Sunday school when we became too big to be forced to attend. The intensity of effort required to prepare for a career can preclude the work needed to maintain skills and knowledge in other fields. The time required for responsible care of family and the duties of being a member of a variety of communities leave few hours for study, meditation, and prayer. We may well find ourselves woefully unprepared to meet the challenges of sickness in ourselves and in others close to us. In our unpreparedness we suffer in our sadness.

Most of us find it difficult, if not nearly impossible, to imagine our death and our disappearance from the world we know. So much of the meaning of our lives is determined by what we do that the thought that we will not be around is frightening, to say the least. What will become of us at the end of life? Donne, in his searing search of himself, asks,

> what's become of man's great extent and proportion, when himself shrinks himself, and consumes himself to a handful of dust? What's become of his soaring thoughts, his compassing thoughts, when himself brings himself to the ignorance, to the thoughtlessness of the grave?[3]

We suffer when we review our life and find obvious failures in purpose and in deed, the fulfilled goals that turned out to be not worth the efforts we made, and the promises and oaths taken and forsaken by us. We look in the mirror and ask, "Who is this person?" These questions we have are spiritual ones, questions that determine our moral stand in our world, pointing to the sources of our spiritual strength, be they religious, philosophical, or simply humanitarian. Our distinctions between good and evil, lines we draw between truth and falsehood, the depth of our acceptance of responsibility for the acts and the commitments we make—all these are spiritual concerns that go far beyond the physical and the emotional components of the self. They classify us in that most interior part of ourselves that we rarely open to the view of others, the life of the spirit. The final question for us in this spiritual search for meaning to our lives is whether we are able to take firm hold of being fully responsible to, and for, the self that we are. The spiritual quest is the awakening of the self in its ambivalence and its need for defining answers to all the questions about that self that will clarify who we are to ourselves and to others.

Modes of Spiritual Suffering

A major source of our suffering from a serious disease is the threat of losing the meaning for our lives. For many of us that meaning is situated in what we do with our bodies: our work, our accomplishments, our families, and our place in our society. Meaning is also closely bound to emotional ties to others. Spiritual suffering is also response to separation: we can feel abandoned by our God, condemned to suffer for no reason obvious to others: we can suffer in the spirit by the realization that our relations with others have been lost, leaving us alone. Difficult and distressing as it is to be ignored by friends or dismissed by family, to feel abandoned by God, stricken with a sickness that brings along with it all of our worst fears and anxieties, can be a humiliating and despairing experience. So much of traditional religion stresses the presence of a loving and caring God, present for us in times of trial; when crises occur that threaten our very existence, there may be a complete collapse of faith when hope for recovery has evaporated. Confirmation of the terrifying reality of feeling forsaken can shatter a religious faith centered on a simple understanding of the spirit of God active in our lives.

Even a most powerful faith, like that of Jesus, can be shaken to its very depth by the feelings of abandonment. The Gospels record the tragic ending of Jesus on the cross when he, in his extremity, quotes from the psalmist, "My God, my God, why have you forsaken me?"[4] This is a profound low point in the life of the spirit, offering us a picture of utter desolation.

A common, almost natural, accompaniment to the conviction that one has been abandoned by God is the haunting fear that illness is retribution, punishment from God for our faulted life. For centuries the debate about theodicy, the justice of God, has continued, obviously without resolution. Human suffering continues as the major stumbling block for faith in a God of justice and of love, and complicates understanding of the human condition in a created order. The human condition—suffering and loss—is, for many, ample evidence for the absence of God. None of us can assert that we have led blameless lives, and certain religious traditions are convinced of the future judgment of a just God that will bode badly for many of us. The torments of a hell are placed in the balance with the glories of a heaven, and for some the onset of a fatal sickness is a this-world beginning of the punishment that God will inflict on sinners. In my experience over the years I have heard many an account that confirms this fear as a reality for some of us.

A contributing factor to a feeling of foreboding that can be a part of the anxiety engendered by concerns about punishment is the recognition that one has ceased any formal adherence to the religious faith of childhood. There can be a sense of guilt in having left the "faith of the fathers" behind, celebrating holy days and seasons as family get-togethers, satisfying the emotional needs of parents and grandparents who still observe them. In speaking with many other professionals, students, and friends I have been impressed with the number of women and men who really do not have any religious foundation to their lives. They are secular Christians and Jews, deriving an ethical basis from the expressed faith of their elders, but claiming none of that faith for themselves. I have heard little in the way of regret or of envy from these persons. There is an outdated quality to many of the traditional religious denominations and faiths of today, suggesting that their beliefs are on a par with a flat earth, a heaven with pearly gates and golden streets, governed by an elderly man with a long gray beard holding court. For many persons educated in the sciences religious concepts are seriously outdated and carry sentimental meaning only, a certain nostalgia for the easy stories of childhood. Some of this suffering that we see is due to a loss that cannot be corrected—the loss of the certainty that there is a center that will hold, a God who will hear and comfort, forgive and accept.

Suffering in the spirit can lead to despondency and depression, arising primarily from the meaninglessness of life now that its end is a distinct possibility. We lose the feeling of being well and happy that Donne reports. "No man is well, that understand not, that values not his being well, that hath not a cheerfulness, and a *joy* in it; and whosoever hath this joy, hath a desire to communicate, to propagate that, which occasions his happiness, and his *joy,* to others."[5] This loss of joy and happiness in the depths of one's being causes us to suffer in the spirit. A feeling that the goals and purposes to which we committed ourselves were not worthy of the price, and an awakening to the reality that there would be no rerun, no second chance to do it the right way, can result in serious loss of the ability to respond positively to any hope offered. It is a commonplace for family, friends, and even caregivers to assume that feeling low and sad is normal with serious disease. Depression is a consequence of loss in the spiritual realm as well as the physical and emotional aspects of the self. Here also, counseling and support are helpful in restoring the person: healing the self, if not curing the body.

In this century we have witnessed the development of psychology as a serious challenger to religion for the soul. In fact, *psyche* is the Greek word for soul, for the spirit within us. Sophisticated schools of thought have developed that place strong emphasis on the unconscious part of our inner selves, that aspect of our personhood we know so poorly, yet comes into the open to surprise, humiliate, humble, and enchant us. Sickness and suffering of the spirit are interpreted by many as being a response to our alienation from our true selves, and from denial of the power of the creative forces that live within our spirits and our minds. We suffer when we do not recognize the power of this spirit to make us whole as persons, even though disease is claiming the body. We suffer when we do not know the conflicts that are a given part of our human personalities. And we suffer when we cannot be healed from the sadness and solitude of sickness, the miseries that the spirit can know when we are isolated from others by disease and by the reactions of others to us as sick persons.

There is a form of suffering in our spirit that can enliven and encourage us when we become ill. This spiritual suffering is the experience we know when we understand the commonality of suffering of all kinds that is the lot of all of us. Seeing the self as a part of all creation, so much of which is in misery and despair, can provide alignment with all others as fellow travelers on a common journey. When we suffer, we are not alone; we have many companions, some of whom have a depth of suffering we will never know. Donne, in his most famous passage in *Devotions Upon Emergent Occasions,* holds us together. In his sickbed he hears the mournful sound of the church bell, signifying the death of someone in the parish. He reflects that,

> No man is an island, entire of itself; every man is a piece of the continent, a part of the main; if a clod be washed away by the sea, Europe is the less, . . . any man's death diminishes me, because I am involved in mankind. . . . [I]f by this consideration of another's danger, I take mine own into contemplation, and so secure myself, by making my recourse to my *God,* who is our only security.[6]

Commentary

In this chapter I have commented upon spiritual suffering, a category of distress and anguish caused by serious illness that is often disregarded in considering the needs of sick people. Surveys done with some regularity vary in their statistics, but show that most persons profess to believe in God, however they might define that reality in their lives. The vagueness of these beliefs might make us question the depth of understanding of the nature and the defining characteristics of the God that is confessed; however, a sense of a spiritual component to both the divine and the mortal being is apparent. And it is this part of us, our spirit, that also suffers when the possibility of death appears.

Whether we interpret our spirit in terms of our unconscious personality that is related to the creator and the created order, or view spirit as a conscious part of our understanding of self and world that is in relation to God through prayer and meditation or through our commitments to all others in love and service matters little. We all have our inner, secret places from which we commune with whatever we choose to support us through our lives. What life means to us will color most clearly our responses to the inevitable crisis that will come when we become sick. How we have chosen our lot, how we are to be with each other, the work that we have done and the promises we have made and kept will establish us in our own eyes and determine the relations we have with the God we have chosen. It is this question of the meaning of life that causes us to suffer when we realize that we have not done what we ought to have done; indeed we have done what we ought not to have done, as an old prayer puts it.

We who care for others when they are very ill, be it personal and family care or the work we do as professional clinicians, must be alert to this hidden spiritual suffering that occurs when disease threatens the very meaning of life before our chosen God. Abandonment, aloneness, despair, and the real possibility of interpretation of disease as divine punishment must be in the minds of those who care for the sick. For many of us, it is the confrontation with the threats of disease that confirms our faith. This spirit of faith may have been a recluse in our hearts for years, but the hazards of living and the clear possibility of dying can awaken it to a God that neither slumbers nor sleeps but awaits our call.

We know that we, and all else that lives, will die. But there is a life of the spirit that places our death in a context of ongoing creativity and purpose. Our acceptance of our death, the sorrow we certainly know at the death of others, and the suffering we must endure are integral parts of the nature of life. There is a cycle of which we are inevitably a part. John Bowker, in the conclusion to his book *The Meanings of Death,* writes,

> It is a human privilege, just as surely as it is a human suffering, to acquire consciously the necessary condition of death, and to affirm it as sacrifice, as the means through which life is enabled and secured. That, consummately, is what Jesus did on the cross. But it is what countless others have also done through the long centuries of human history.[7]

God, in the many and varied ways that our sense of the divine is envisioned, has been known to us through history in what we call spirit. Intangible, yet present; heard in the heart, yet not seen; a spirit defining of our own spirit, giving meaning to all life.

Notes

1. Ezek. 37:14 NRSV.
2. John Donne, *The Complete Poetry and Selected Prose of John Donne,* ed. Charles M. Coffin (New York: Modern Library, 1994), 415.
3. Ibid., 420.
4. Mark 15:34 NRSV.
5. Donne, *The Complete Poetry and Selected Prose,* 426.
6. Ibid., 441.
7. John Bowker, *The Meanings of Death* (New York: Cambridge University Press, 1991), 227.

8

"I Still Have to Shop"

Samuel Johnson, the renowned critic, poet, dictionary compiler, and conversationalist of eighteenth-century England, said, "It matters not how a man dies, but how he lives. The act of dying is not of importance, it lasts so short a time."[1] While it is no longer a truism that dying lasts a short time, still the defining times of our lives are the lived ones. And these times are experiences that medical students can learn about as they anticipate their future years caring for seriously ill persons. The hopes and the expectations of students that they will be caring and compassionate, attentive to the specific needs of individuals for whom they are responsible, can only be realized if they learn to listen to the needs of their patients. These needs go far beyond specific treatments and diagnostic studies: they include understanding the daily living styles and requirements of their patients. There are no general check-lists of the personal needs we have for our day-by-day lives other than food, clothing, and, for most of us, affection and companionship.

The diagnosis of a serious disease such as cancer, kidney failure, or AIDS brings with it the distinct possibility of a threat to one's life. Recognition of this can be devastating, an announcement we hoped we would never hear. Anxiety and fear become instant companions.

But, when the initial shock has subsided somewhat, there is the real-ization that the mundane demands of life are still operative. Shopping and laundry must be done, civic responsibilities are still present, the bills must be paid, and the house cleaned. However, patients usually enter a new phase in their lives, one that includes reflection on pre-vious goals and purposes, redefinition of relationships and commit-ments, and an awakening to parts of their lives perhaps ignored and undervalued in the past. These aspects of the life of a person with a serious disease must be concerns of the caring physician and they can only be learned from the patient, that individual who has as many and as diverse needs and hopes as the physician.

We can never really know what another person feels since each of us is an individual with unique genetic, familial, psychological, and experiential qualities. But we can come close to an approximation of that knowing by hearing the story of each patient and attempting to locate ourselves, for the moment at least, in the place of the other. This is more easily said than done, since careful listening requires time and attention. But it has its rewards: the listener can receive, through conversations with patients, a self-knowledge that is rewarding, although perhaps uncomfortable in its acquisition. This learning about the self of the caregiver—with revelations and a new self-understanding—can be one of the richest rewards for caring for others. But before this can happen we must be able to meet the patient at the place where this special individual is at this moment—newly diagnosed with a serious disease.

Ms. A. was lying in the hospital bed in a room shared with another woman. She had been feeling sick for several weeks, becoming weak and pale, and finally developed a fever. She was hospitalized, tests were done, and she was waiting, with considerable anxiety, for the results. Her doctor appeared at the door, came into the room, and stood at the foot of her bed with arms folded on his chest. He said, "You have leukemia and I will have to see what kind of treatment to give you." As he said these words, and turned to leave the room, her sick roommate reached across the great distance that suddenly separated her from the rest of the world at this moment, took her hand, and held it tightly.

This is a very sad anecdote, a dismal account of abandonment and disregard of another person at a moment of wrenching need. If there ever was a time, in the history of the world, for the touch of a doctor's hand, it was at that moment of giving the bad news. We can very easily and quickly blame this thoughtless physician for his heartless behavior. In fact, this type of patient "care" is exactly what medical students want to learn to avoid and convert that time into a deeply experienced encounter between two human beings at an instant of need and near despair.

Many persons, both within and outside the healthcare professions, write about and speak to the need for physicians to learn to talk with their patients about the personal aspects of their diseases: the implications of their sickness for their life. But inability to converse easily and in depth with other persons about serious issues in their lives is common among us, and certainly not limited to doctors. Lawyers, clergy, and many others have the same problems when it comes to speaking to intensely personal concerns. Indeed, many of us as spouses, parents, and adult children balk at confiding secrets, revealing doubts and fears, and disclosing those innermost parts of ourselves that we know will prove us to be less than we want others to believe us to be. Because of our hesitancy and our lack of training, many physicians are completely at a loss when it comes to talking about what a serious disease means for the patient. Just asking the questions becomes a major hurdle, to say nothing of the difficulties in discussing the implications of the disease for the intimate parts of life.

This is the point at which the patient can teach us the skills of speaking to what seem to be monumental and overwhelming personal issues. At times of severe stress that threaten our very existence, a strain is placed upon the structures in our lives, the foundations that we say we depend on to see us through rough encounters. Marriage is one of the supports that are considered important in times of difficulty. But the nature of the relationship, not the marriage contract, will define the support. For some, the burdens and the dangers of serious sickness undo a relationship that has seemed comfortable and normal.

Mr. B. is sixty-five years of age and retired from a retail business. Four years ago he was diagnosed with colon cancer, had surgery, and now wears a colostomy bag. He did well after his original treatment until nine months ago when it was found that the cancer had spread to his liver. His response to chemotherapy is disappointing; he seems to feel fairly well, although nausea and drowsiness are constant companions. He is married to an anxious woman who refuses to come with him to the oncology clinic because the place makes her "nervous." He appears lonely and is delighted to talk with other patients and the staff, seeking assurances that he is an accepted part of the group of patients and not alone during this formidable experience. Most of the patients in the clinic have a spouse, an adult child, a close friend or neighbor with them for transportation, for conversation, getting a cup of coffee, or just being there watching television together to pass the time.

What seems, at first glance, to be a form of abandonment or neglect of her husband's very real and apparent needs may suggest further assessment and attention by the staff. Arnold Feldman, M.D., a psychiatrist at the University of Pennsylvania, writes,

> The spouse or significant other of the terminally ill patient is experiencing anguish that, although different from the agony of the patient, may be every bit as painful. At the same time that the spouse is faced with the loss of a healthy mate and the anticipation of the death of the spouse, she or he is usually serving as the primary caregiver. The spouse's coping mechanisms are being tested to their fullest, just at the time she or he is required to function in a most competent and autonomous way.[2]

The wife of the man with colon cancer may well have nearly overwhelming feelings of anxiety about the immediate future; she may be angry at her husband, and then startled by the guilt that that anger engenders. The stress is intensified by the prospect of loss of an intimate companion, a sadness complicated by grief at approaching abandonment.

The admission that one could experience rage at the approaching death of a spouse is, of course, startling and a source of further embarrassment, shame, and sorrow. If, as in many marriages, there is ambivalence about the emotional content and depth of the relationship, resentment at dependence, and a history of strife and disagreement, feelings of guilt and shame are intensified and hurtful. In relationships where love has been a powerful adhesive force, the sense of loss can approach the unbearable. All these feelings, so many of them carrying mixed and powerful overtones, can be learned by students as they pursue their goal of becoming a caring and sensitive physician. In fact, one of the challenges for caregivers is learning to explore and understand the vast range of feelings that we can know, these emotions and responses that we catch a glimpse of in our work with patients. John Hinton, in the *Experience of Illness,* writes,

> Dying people experience a series of losses and foresee yet more. . . .
> Separation has already begun and some people or places will never
> be seen again. . . . So grief is appropriate to those who recognize
> they are dying. Particular aspects of life have now finished forever.
> . . . At times their sense of loss can bring deep regret and pain. But
> a sense of peace or pleasure may attend the recognition that some
> struggles and unpleasant features of living have now ceased; so bal-
> anced against the sense that the remaining sources of enjoyment are
> reduced and finite may be a relief that, say, a lonely life of continued
> ill-health need not be endured much longer.[3]

We differ in the ways we organize our defenses when we are confronted by the possibility of catastrophe. When the initial shock of the diagnosis of a life-threatening disease is somewhat dissipated, and plans are made for treatment, some patients turn the control of the course of the disease—its therapies and ongoing laboratory and evaluative procedures and studies—completely over to the doctors. After all, the physicians and the technicians know best about what should be done and have the appropriate skills and knowledge to do it well. There are many patients, however, who do not let control slip out of their hands. Knowing the fallibility we all are subject to, and the potential for harm if errors occur in memory or in calculations, many patients keep accurate records. Mr. C. recorded all of his laboratory data in a diary that dated back to the day of his original diagnosis of acute leukemia. Intelligent and successful in business, he and his wife quickly learned the medical and scientific aspects of his disease and the various treatment options available to them. They assessed the medical facilities available and chose the one they thought best for them. The clinic and hospital staffs quickly learned that this couple knew as much as, if not more than, many of them about leukemia and its treatment. In these times of easy access via electronic media, being informed is a simple task.

The significance of this approach to one's sickness is considerable, and the medical students recognized this when Mr. C. and his wife came to class to talk about their experiences. There were occasional humorous moments when he was tempted to sermonize and offer generalities about the history of his illness and the practice of medicine. His wife was quick to interrupt, gently but accurately, correcting him and letting us know that she was a partner in the progressive history of her husband's life. The students were in awe of them and their quiet affirmation that they were doing all that could be done in this time and place to confront the reality of a very serious illness. An important lesson for the students was seeing and hearing that day an example of the best type of patient they could expect in the future: one who was a willing, intelligent, and competent partner in the management of a serious sickness. Impressive also was the potent reminder that the good physician must know as much as can be known about the diseases that present themselves to us in persons seeking help.

Severe tests are presented to families when serious disease levels husband or wife. Current therapy for some persons with leukemia involves a bone-marrow transplant. Before this is done, intensive chemotherapy is given until the disease is in remission. This experience, usually associated with loss of hair, nausea and vomiting, and extended hospitalization, is exhausting and traumatic following, as it does, upon learning the diagnosis and the very real possibilities for disastrous consequences. After a person has received a marrow transplant, there is a period of time—weeks to months—when the patient can have no close contact with any other person because the normal blood cells and immune system that protect us from infectious germs have not reached functional levels. During hospitalization and after returning home, there are restrictions that are profound. The patient can have no physical contact with others—spouse, children, friends: no kisses, shaking hands, or even touching. Sexual intimacy is not permitted. A mask must be worn when out in public or near anyone with even the mildest cold. Fresh fruits and vegetables may have germs on them and cannot be allowed in the house. The bathroom must be kept immaculate with daily cleansing and sanitizing. It takes little imagination to grasp the impact of all this upon Mrs. D., a twenty-seven-year-old woman with two children, ages three and five. Not only has she suffered through the anxieties of learning that she has leukemia, a fatal disease; aspects of her life so central to her definition of herself as a wife, a lover, a mother, a friend, and a citizen must be suspended for a long time without assurance that the therapy will succeed.

A separation from one's world this intense calls upon the inventive and insightful skills of her caregivers to provide the support and the encouragement, the cheer and the confidence that only a true sense of identification with her can offer. This collection of interpersonal skills can be learned by the students from this young woman and patients like her. She is the teacher of us as we learn the terrors of separation, the anxieties associated with future dire possibilities, the sad feelings of not being with and for the others so central to how we define ourselves to ourselves and to others. We are humbled before her courage, and we understand the power of love to support the sacrifice of our own wishes and desires before the requirements of others. Receiving this revelation of the needs of others that we can help satisfy can be a most rewarding aspect of caring for others.

There are social components to medical care, all too obvious to us in our time. The number of persons for whom health care is essentially not accessible is alarming. This is an era when severe economic and time restrictions by insurers make the type and the quality of medical services questionable for many persons. The implications of present policies are of import to healthcare providers; they can also be alarming to the poor, the uninsured, and those with certain inherited or chronic diseases.

Mrs. E. is a first-generation Italian-American woman in her forties, married to a day laborer with no medical insurance. She is obese and sits quietly in the clinic, giving the distinct impression of a submissive, passive, and pleasant person who would not want to bother anyone. For a year she has seen blood in her bowel movements. Only recently has she noticed some dizziness and weakness associated with an unexpected loss of weight. She finally went to see a doctor in her neighborhood because she had no means of transportation; he sent her immediately to the hospital where colon cancer with metastases was easily diagnosed. She was referred to the outpatient chemotherapy clinic and treatment begun. Her obvious passivity and seeming stoic acceptance of the desperate nature of her sickness alarmed the nurses managing her treatment. Consultation with the social worker, arrangement for Medicaid payments and transportation on a community van placed her in a strange new locus in her life. She found herself surrounded and protected by the medical center clinic staff who became as a family for her. Here were persons to whom she was important; her welfare was their obvious and devoted concern. She began to attend to herself as a woman; she talked with staff about her daily life and her hopes, smiled, and entered into the communal life of the clinic. She commented, with obvious pleasure, that even the van driver asked how she was doing, yet another one who cared. There was a sad, yet triumphant, note in her observation to the medical student that "getting cancer may have been the best thing in my life."

She taught her student the importance of social context in interpreting the impact of illness on the life of a specific individual. She showed so clearly in her own developing life that there are parts to our existence that do not fit a simplistic pathophysiological understanding of disease. We are persons who can change and grow if assistance is given in freeing another to become what is possible, given all our limitations. Windows can be opened and the fresh air of new experience can cheer us. Even in dying, one may find life for the first time. Awakening to a new morning can be a metaphor with deep significance for one who is facing the end.

When it becomes apparent that the available and standard means of treatment have been exhausted and there is little ahead but palliative care, experimental protocols may be suggested and accepted or declined, based upon individual choice and the personal and family environment. It is at these times that the depth and significance of close relationships becomes so clear and revealing of the life that has been lived up to this hour. For the student this is a key learning point about the role of the physician in care of the dying. The words that patients use can be loaded with meaning, fitting closely to observation of behavior.

Mr. F., a delightful man in his late sixties, had come to the end of useful chemotherapy for his leukemia. His bone marrow was not recovering from the last round of treatment and he was slowly fading. He seemed as cheerful as ever, coming to clinic with his wife, hand in hand. They are a smiling couple, speaking easily with staff and other patients. But today the student notes a subtle change. In the past, they often spoke of their next trip to see their daughter and grandchildren, their plans to go south for a few weeks in the depth of winter, or some approaching holiday gathering. Today they speak in the past tense; they have had a good life together raising a family, enjoying friends, understanding the significance of the intimacy they have shared over all these years. They have shared about as much of life as it is possible to do, and now the ending is in sight.

It is apparent to the student that an acceptance has been accomplished, a tacit agreement to await the ending, a clear acknowledgment of a life—a good life—coming to a close. Further management of the care of this couple will be accurately influenced by this observation and a shift to new and altered needs of the patient and his wife as they sit and smile and talk. The student pays attention.

A major learning experience for the students is awareness of the living styles and communication methods patients use for talking about themselves, their needs, their relationships, and their idiosyncratic ways of dealing with the unexpected and frightening events that descend upon their lives. Being told that one has a serious medical condition that could be a threat to life often causes us to ask, "Why me?" This is often followed by a pervasive sense of isolation, of feeling very alone, surrounded by a circle of healthy people pursuing their daily lives as if all was well. This feeling of separation from others can be accentuated by the changes in appearance due to surgery, X-ray treatment, and chemotherapy. Loss of hair can be very bothersome to both women and men; it is such an obvious change in one's appearance, noticeable to all. The men put on a baseball cap and the women resort to turbans and wigs. These become, in the clinic setting, an identification badge, as it were, allowing rapid recognition of one's fellow patients. The setting of a chemotherapy clinic in a large room where the patients are together can be most comforting: the patients get to know each other and share common experiences and modes of dealing with the exigencies of this new and restricting life.

Not only do the patients get to know each other, but they soon develop friendships. Not only serious topics are discussed. There is a certain humor that develops as the rigors of treatment and the ups and downs of the courses of their illnesses proceed. There is also a strong sense of community and support that holds the patients together, often to a depth that surprises them. A student writes,

> It's Halloween today, and the nurses in the chemotherapy clinic seem determined to observe the occasion. They have put up orange and black streamers across every wall and are wearing pointy black hats which wobble from side to side as they set up the IV stands. . . . Mr. F. is sixty-eight years old and he is dying. They told him about his colon cancer four years ago. . . . He began chemotherapy and the doctors were pleased with his progress. Then things began to go downhill. Current chemotherapy was failing and his tumor had spread to his lungs. . . .
>
> Today there was depressing news. Another man's tumor had grown larger despite the latest new drug. Now Eddie speaks up. At thirty-one, he knows he appears out of place in this clinic. In fact, another patient told him the first day he came in, "What are you doing here? You're too young to have cancer." Eddie seemed to think he would beat the disease, even when the doctors told him the tumor was inoperable; he continued to believe it would just go away. One of the nurses is talking to Mr. F. as she draws blood for the third time. "Everyone seems so jolly today," she says quietly.

"We're always jolly," replies Mr. F. "Why shouldn't we be? The thing is, none of us chose to have this disease. But we can't lament it, either. We're just lucky to be alive. I may die tomorrow or I may die in twenty years. But until then, I'm gonna make sure I damn well live my life."[4]

I have watched a group of four men with colon cancer develop an amazing relationship, in concert with their wives, at the chemotherapy clinic that they attend each Thursday. Storytelling and joking characterize their hours at the clinic; they are also very attentive to any one of their little group that seems out of sorts. But they do exhibit an infectious humor that keeps their lives in a healthy perspective of reality. They are also quick to share with each other any "tricks of the trade" that make dealing with the problems of cancer and its treatments a bit easier.

On one of the days when I was in clinic recruiting patient-teachers for the course, I was asked by the women volunteers what I was doing as I went around talking with patients. Was I doing a survey? It was the day of the week when the patients were mostly women with breast cancer, and the volunteers who offered coffee, a bagel, and easy conversation were women who, themselves, had had cancer of the breast. I showed them the information sheet that patients receive; when they read the title of the course, Seminar on the Seriously Ill Patient, they immediately criticized me for that label. They had had cancer, had recovered, and thought that I was overemphasizing the hazards of the disease. I was obviously quite surprised, but pleased and impressed by their positive approach to what I still consider a "serious" disease. When, in a counterresponse, I asked one of the volunteers what she did in the clinic, she told me the following story.

A woman in her early thirties, for whom English was her second language, had just been told that the biopsy of her breast showed cancer, and a mastectomy was the treatment of choice. She was visibly shocked, and not sure that she understood what all this would mean for her. The volunteer, after observing the inept response of the doctor, said, "Come with

me." They went into an examining room where the volunteer unbut-
toned her blouse and, smiling, said, "This is what you will look like." The
young woman also smiled, was obviously relieved and reassured by what
she saw, and they returned to the clinic setting together.

Another young woman posed a different and more difficult task
for communication with her student.

She was in her thirties, a slender, frail black woman with an impassive
face and subdued voice. She sat quietly in clinic, spoke to no other patients,
and was withdrawn from the social atmosphere. She had metastatic colon
cancer and her treatments were not going well. Both of her parents had
died within the past year and she had no siblings or spouse. The student
was overwhelmed by the tragedy of the story, its loneliness and sense of
near despair. She was distressed by her inability to engage her patient-
teacher in any meaningful dialogue and felt herself a failure in such a
simple task. As we talked in the seminar, it reminded us that there are
times when we appear to be powerless to assist, to effect change, to offer
hope. The depth of personal emotional emptiness being lived out by this
patient became clear, and the need for intensive treatment—both psycho-
logical and pharmacological—of her depression was obvious.

Comment

In this chapter I have presented some of the mundane aspects of
being sick with a serious, even life-threatening, disease. All of the
concerns about illness are not limited to diagnosis and medical and
surgical treatments, obviously important as they are. But we all,
regardless of circumstances, have daily lives in families, communities,
workplaces, and in our interior selves. If we are going to provide the
quality of care that we know is important and humane, then we must
know about the daily lives that our patients live out and how the caregivers can enhance those lives. We can learn from patients what their
specific priorities are, what exterior resources they have or lack, what
inner supports they call upon in religion, art, music, literature, and

other creative aspects of our common life that we should know about. A key factor for students of medicine and other health professions is a willingness to learn of these things so that we can offer the best and fullest comprehension of the individual life that is possible for persons facing the trials of serious illness.

The most reliable source for this information is the patient, resident in the body that has betrayed its owner by becoming sick and presenting the possibility of ultimate loss. The gains from learning about those personal lives and adventures is immeasurable, and finally, of great help to the patient. Only the patient knows the story of the life that is endangered; only the patient can, when confidence has been confirmed, tell the little and big secrets that have added to the value of that life. Patients honor us with their stories and their accounts of the defining events of their lives. We, in gratitude for their narratives, assure confidentiality and use our wits as best we can to provide the best care possible for another person whom we honor. The patient is the source of the ongoing growth and maturation of the physician, the nurse, and other caregivers, even family and friends. Patients teach us the meanings of suffering, endurance, humor, and faith in our lives. We know that we shall, at some future date, be in the same situation as our patients are today. There is a saying attributed to one John Bradford who saw a man on the way to the gallows: "But for the grace of God there goes John Bradford."[5] I think it takes little imagination for us to replace his name with ours when we care for the seriously ill.

Notes

1. J. Boswell, *Boswell's Life of Johnson*, vol. 2, ed. by George Birkbeck Hill (Oxford: Clarendon Press, 1887), 106–107.

2. A. Feldman, "The Dying Patient," *Psychiatric Clinics of North America* 10, no. 1 (March 1987): 103.

3. J. Hinton, "Coping with Terminal Illness," *The Experience of Illness* (London: Tavistock Publications, 1984), 235.

4. M. Salameh, personal communication, 1996.

5. J. Bartlett, *Familiar Quotations,* 15th ed., ed. Emily M. Beck (Boston: Little, Brown, 1980), 162.

9

"I Learned How to Listen"

The central learning experience for medical students in the Seminar on the Seriously Ill Patient is *listening* to a patient, paying careful attention to what is being said to us by another person who is sick. This may seem to be an obvious, even simplistic, task for anyone caring for sick persons, but it is not; patients often comment on the difficulties they encounter in trying to tell their stories—their "histories"—to their doctors. Are the personal concerns of the patient unimportant? Are they too intimate, too individualistic to be relevant to the pressing medical problems presented by cancer, kidney failure, AIDS, devastating accidents, or the host of other crises in our lives? What are the experiences of students as they talk with their patient-teachers?

The Patient as a Person

Although it seems apparent, even at first glance, students learn that patients are persons. Of course, they know this as a fact, a visible and accepted aspect of being a human being. But so much of their premedical education and their information about medicine as a profes-

129

sion has to do with persons as patients, as people who are sick or disabled in one way or another and seeking help from physicians in offices, clinics, and hospitals. Patients are often referred to by diagnosis rather than by name, and the details of their personal lives are considered as interesting, perhaps, but not crucial to the management of the disease. When students without any clinical experience sit down and ask patients how things are going with them, they begin a new chapter in their education. What, in other circumstances, seem like ordinary interpersonal skills of conversation about daily living, can, in professional settings, seem difficult at best, overwhelming at worst. The students ask me, "What do I say to my patient? How can I possibly talk to someone so sick when I don't know anything about them or their disease? Should I look up their disease in a textbook?" At our early sessions we discuss these issues and I can reassure the students that their teachers are quite adept at putting them at ease and moving the conversation right along.

The fifty-year-old nun with metastatic breast cancer, mentioned earlier, confessed to her student that she had been mistaken when she thought that the loss of a breast would be less devastating to her than to another woman, since there was no man in her life. Also, having worn a habit for years did not prevent the shock of the loss of her hair. She said, "A good physician listens very carefully to the patient and respects the patient's knowledge of her body." She had gone to her doctor when she had back pain (her first symptom of breast cancer spread to her spine); she was assured that it was just stress, and was advised to take a vacation. She commented on the indignity of being ordered to strip before a group of doctors on rounds, talked about her anger at being so sick so soon, her depression and her bargaining with God. She talked with her student about the importance of the simplest of human acts: "A touch on the shoulder can make the difference between improvement and not." In a situation like this, students are quick to hear the message of the hope for sensitivity to simple needs and gentle ways from their caregivers. Patients are persons like us with emotions and concerns common to all. Learning to listen and attend to those concerns and feelings are the tasks and the joys of the profession. Based upon our own unique experiences and personalities, we have expectations of how healthcare professionals should behave toward us, and how the healthcare system should function. When these expectations are not met, there is palpable dissatisfaction.

The student's teacher was being treated for recurrent cancer of the cervix; he sat with her and they talked. Her treatment was a routine protocol, but for her it was everything. It would be easy, in light of the uncomplicated nature of her treatment, to lose sight of how she saw herself with cancer. "I just tried to be there for her to talk to, and I came away from our conversations with an understanding of what it's like to be dealing with pain, extended disability, the stigma of having cancer, and mortality. I hope I can keep that knowledge on file."

The patient as a person is usually a member of a family that responds in varied ways to the jarring diagnosis of a disease that threatens life. Patients teach us about the relevance of family for them and how we must be awake to the functions families fulfill for care. Serious disease can highlight the protective and supportive functions of a structured family; it can also provide the wedge that drives persons apart because of the stresses induced by the threat of death.

The mentor for the student was a woman in her thirties dying of lymphoma. After spending weeks meeting with her, the student said, "I learned that the most important thing in the relationship was honesty." Her teacher talked about her shock at abandonment by her boyfriend, and her need to move back to her old home for support. The student said, "My teacher made me acutely aware of the fragility of family structure in a medical crisis, and how you have to treat the family, not just the patient. I wouldn't have thought of that before taking the course." The patient is a person, but also a person in a larger context of family, community, and world in which the doctor participates as a major player in the drama of a life.

How to Listen, How to Talk

As medical students we are taught that the diagnosis of a disease is derived from a history of the patient carefully elicited by a trained doctor; the purpose of the physical examination is to confirm that diagnosis. If this is so, then listening to the patient is most important. We must learn to listen in a critical way, alert to nuances in speech, to inconsistencies in the narrative, hints of events, experiences, or relationships that could be crucial to understanding the present problems of this person. As many of us know from daily contacts with others—family, close friends, associates—we often hold back on communicating negative feelings, anger, words that might be hurtful or demeaning of ourselves. In talking with patients, the personal setting must be such as to allow, even encourage, conversation that is completely open and revealing of the life of the patient. The caregiver must be an active listener, positively engaged in the story being told by the patient. It is important to recall that, although patient and doctor appear to have the same goal—relief of symptoms and return of health—the ways they see both the goals and the ways to achieve them may be quite divergent. We must hear the story the patient has to tell.

One student, just before meeting his patient-teacher for the first time, commented later, "I had no idea what to say. I thought I would have to be profound, or cry." Fortunately, the patients are forewarned of the anxiety of the students, and are quick to set them at ease. This patient, Bob, was dying slowly of an ill-defined viral disease, getting sicker each week, finally confined to bed at home in the care of his wife, a nurse. The student and I visited him a few days before his death; the student told Bob that he had written a paper about their experiences and what he had learned. They shook hands and thanked each other for what they had done for each other. Bob reached to hug his student and said, "You allowed me to do something with the last days of my life—to offer a gift out of my hopelessness." The student went on to be chief resident in obstetrics and gynecology; he said, "I'm still learning as a doctor, but my real education began with Bob."

Listening with an ear sensitive to both the patient and the self as questioner is an informing experience that will be a determinant in care for the sick. There are amazing differences in national, religious, social, and sociomedical-cultural patterns in the patient population. There is considerable uniformity among physicians in the United States in terms of social class, economic security, education level, and such determinants as having a physician as a parent or close relative. These characteristics can be an impressive barrier separating doctor from hospital and clinic patients. Learning to listen without prejudice or bias toward another is essential to providing compassionate care; while we are loath to admit our own prejudices, we know they exist. To ensure that they do not interfere with care, we must develop empathy for the sick and sad and an understanding of the self that keeps us open to the reality of the impact of serious disease on persons. Again, only an openness of the self in contact with the sick and the suffering can give us the courage to abandon our prejudices. Accepting others as worthy and needy of our care is a powerful determinant of the quality, both of that care and of the caregiver.

In our contemporary world, certain diseases, mental and physical conditions, and personal behaviors are rejected and despised, and labeled unacceptable, abnormal, or sick. For a decade after its appearance in the United States AIDS was such a condition. Originally associated with male homosexuality, and later with intravenous drug use, AIDS carried a highly charged aura that was a determinant in medical and social care. It is terrifying to have a disease considered fatal; to also be an outcast from society can be a frightful added burden. Some of the best teachers in the seminar are AIDS patients. They are usually younger than cancer patients; it can be discomfiting for students to speak with persons their own age who are dying. But there is that revelation, that sure knowledge that this is another human being who, often in despair, is seeking help and comfort. Our behavior is controlled by that knowledge.

The student's teacher was a young man with AIDS. One day he was taken to the emergency room where the student found him frightened, withdrawn, curled up in the fetal position; the student said, "I reached

out and touched him, and he stopped shaking; he wasn't so scared any-
more. It was as if I had given him a cup of water and a pill. I don't
think you can get much more graphic than that." Again, the touch of
the human hand is a sign of attention, of personal feeling, of sympathy.

As a play on the word, I would mention "patient." One of the
learned skills that are picked up by students is that of acquiring
patience. This is a personality trait that can be learned from patients
as they move, predictably, on that road that has no returning, the
road to death. They teach us patience in the daily routines of diagnostic tests, treatments, the seemingly endless waiting for results and
for improvement in health. A student's "fiction," based upon her
patient-teacher's story, tells us,

> But the one truly unbearable thing—if I had to pick just one—is
> being made to wait. My moments are slipping away from me and
> yet I must wait minutes, hours, entire mornings and afternoons in
> the treatment room, with its dull tiles and fluorescent lights and
> everywhere you turn TV screens and vacant, resigned patients. The
> other day a fresh-faced student, visiting with one of the other cancer
> victims, told me she'd see me next week. That broke me down com-
> pletely. "Oh my dear," I said, wanting to laugh or cry. "I only live
> one day at a time." And then I did, I put my face in my hands and
> wept.[1]

We also learn patience in the foibles and the unintentional hurts and
errors of others that patients relate.

Another facet of medical care that fascinates, even as it annoys,
caregivers is the problem of the "bad" patient, the one who tells us
to go away and leave them alone, refuses to have the X-ray taken now,
tells us how bad the hospital is run, and wants to go home. These
persons are so different from the "good" patient who is compliant,
friendly, and cheerful even in the face of bad news, and so thankful
for all that has been done for them. The "bad" patient is a trial, but
tells us something of the role of mind and spirit in helping heal, pal-
liate, and occasionally cure. In ways not well understood, there are

emotional and psychological aspects to healing that are strong and desirable and seem related to the abilities of some persons to take impressive control of their lives and what happens to them when there are various options offered. Often, to the confusion of the staff, the "bad" patients do better, suggesting that we do have influences upon our health that are not limited to medications and surgery.

The students also learn to be patient in their eliciting the life stories of others. As I noted earlier, medical students mislabel the seminar, calling it a course on "death and dying." Their initial expectation is that their patient-teachers are concerned about the possibility, indeed the imminence, of their death and will speak to it. They are surprised to find that concerns are for living and not about dying. A student writes,

> It seems strange now, looking back, that when I met him he only had six months to live. Every Thursday he would come to clinic sporting his hat of the week—usually a baseball cap from an obscure Western Connecticut little league team; or a brown plaid fisherman's hat on cold days. . . . We spent little time talking about how things were going with John's health—I'd always ask how the previous week had gone, and would always receive the same smiling response, "Can't complain!"—followed by Susan's urging him to tell me how things *really* were. John wasn't really a talker, but he was most certainly a liver. . . .
>
> I realized over time that their feelings for me and interest in my life was as much medicine for them as the strongest chemotherapy. That if *not* talking about sickness was how they dealt with things, that that was okay too. . . . I do worry about Susan who has always been the giving one—that people have grown to depend on her in that role, and have erased the concept of Susan as needing from their minds.[2]

The students learn to be patient, and to wait for their teachers to raise the inevitable topic of death, the event that we all will know. We must be patient in our talk with the seriously ill, allowing them to, in due time, raise the questions whose answers we do not know. One of the discoveries that students have is the support that their patient-teachers provide as they struggle to learn how to listen and learn about what it means to be so sick. Most patients that I have spoken with are eager to help medical students learn, and are quite "patient" with their students in their task of overcoming their anxieties. One student noted that, "Not only did my patient have her own life, resources, support, and self-esteem, but she also supported me in my ineptness and unease more than I could support her."

How Do We Face Death?

There is an almost imperceptible movement toward friendship with patients who are very sick, and this relationship can induce very mixed feelings. One student, noting the odd coincidence of her patient-teacher dying in the hospital yet speaking of her hopes and desires for living, found this painful and confusing. Another alarming concern of the student was her negative reaction to the physical wasting of her teacher: the dry, cracked lips; the nauseated expression on her face; the grogginess from medication. The student found this puzzling and was distressed to realize that the appearance of her teacher, instead of producing compassion and thereby deepening their developing friendship, created a feeling of isolation. The student retreated emotionally and saw the woman as a patient in need of help, no longer as a teacher of the art of dying. Even more distressing was the recognition by the student that her patient-teacher was acutely aware of her altered reaction. This type and quality of introspection is the beginning of the learning process leading to being with, and for, our patients as they suffer and die. This is one of the milestones on the road to being a physician that must be recognized, and proper support offered to encourage the ongoing discovery of the self and finding the ways to convert the anxiety and the doubt into assurance that we will accompany our patients all the way.

Dying and death are difficult and painful topics to discuss, even with healthy people. Obviously, no one knows anything about what death will bring to us. Religion and philosophy have much to say on the matter, but there is no evidence that we can offer to comfort the seriously ill who are dying, with one exception. And that is our promise that, as their life closes, they will not be abandoned. It seems that most persons are fully aware of the fact of death, the certainty that all life ends. The stumbling block for many of us is our fear that we will die alone; the very unwelcome vision of being alone in a hospital room at the end of the corridor with no other person to comfort us as we die. The medical student writes about visiting his patient-teacher in the hospital:

> All I was thinking was, "Go home, Rose. You ought to go home." My patient Rose from my seminar on the seriously ill. She has metastatic ovarian cancer. . . . I thought maybe Rose would have some doubts about seeing me . . . some people get embarrassed when they're sick. It was dim. Yes, dim, but not so dim that I could not see the changes in Rose. Her eyes were sunk, and her arms so skinny, and no more wig—just a strange white turban to cover her naked head, and a strange blue nightgown, and a few tubes, and what looked like the broken-off end of an Atari 2600 joystick clipped to the front of her costume. . . . Rose was tired. "So many doctors and nurses, and people bothering me all the time. I know they mean well," she said. Then let slip, "I know you mean well." She wanted me to leave but I didn't have the heart.
> "I'm happy to see you have your own room, a little privacy," I tried. But I'm remembering, Rose never liked all the privacy she had. An orphan's privacy, a divorcee's privacy, an assembly-line worker's privacy. No, what I called privacy, Rose might call loneliness. That's the difference, I guess.[3]

This type of personal narrative is available to us as we talk with patients and certainly informs any planning management for the final days. Again, it is the patient who instructs us about what can and must be done, what is expected of caregivers.

How do we discuss death and the way we die with patients? It is a topic that requires ingenuity and sensitivity to the many nuances we apply to delicate and personal issues of our lives, and the lives of those close to us. Again, there are many individualized styles for both discussing and actually facing the prospect of death, and the patient is

the teacher here. One of the key principles of conversation is applic-
able here also: we must send the message to patients, both directly
and indirectly, that we are available, interested, and committed to
assuring the best of care as death approaches. This means being alert
to those signals that are sent out to see if we are interested in talking
about the various concerns patients have, especially what is to be
done when nothing more can be done. Questions, anecdotes,
phrases, quotations—all tip off the caregivers to what the concerns
are. The medical students are astounded at the variety of perspectives
that patients have about their own condition. One patient-teacher
with metastatic breast cancer absolutely confounded her student by
her assertion that she did not know why she was in an oncology
clinic; her doctor told her she needed this treatment, and she
accepted his advice, but was unable to say why she was there. As
might be expected, this patient posed an enormous challenge to a
young student trying to learn how to care for seriously ill patients.

One of the ways we care for persons is allowing them to determine their lives. This may require alterations in certain protocols for
treatment, changing schedules and appointment times, offering
options to treat and not to treat. There are many perspectives on
dying, and we are to be alert to the needs of the patient, not the
wishes of the physicians. One way of "dying" that is a source of terror
for many of us is the condition of dementia, the loss of the mind.
Most commonly seen now in Alzheimer's disease, it is also seen in
AIDS, usually as a late development, but not necessarily. For many
persons, this possibility of being alive but without a mind is worse
than death. The provision of proper care is severely compounded
when there is the obvious loss of personhood before physical death.

Patients help us to demystify death, to see the event as the
inevitable final stage of a lived life.

*He was a contractor, a heavyset and strong man quietly proud of a life
spent working hard, raising a good family, and being a conservative
and respected member of his community. He was diagnosed with
leukemia and did well for a while, finally coming to the end of available treatment. Not expecting to meet in him a person with an active*

and artistic imagination, I was surprised and delighted to listen to his
account of a dream or a vision that he had one night in the hospital. As
he lay in his bed there appeared before him a tree with its limbs bare.
Lovely in outline against the sky, he pondered its significance. Even as he
watched, leaves appeared on the tree, branch by branch until it was a
glorious announcement of spring. With quiet confidence he explained
that this was the image, the concept, the revelation of the event of his
death. It was merely the first act of a drama that would be glorious and
renewing.

One of the functions that caregivers can offer is the opportunity
to help patients review their lives and evaluate them, search out the
relationships, the accomplishments that define that life, and look to
the possibility of a good death in competent hands. These goals can
be the combined effort of the patient and the talented caregiver
awake to the need we all have for bringing life to a proper close.

What Do Patients Want?

When we listen to patients talk about themselves and their lives, we
learn the idiosyncrasies so essential to their proper and personal care.
What does an individual person want from those who provide that
care? What are the specifics of this singular person, this one-of-a-kind
family that must be known so that attention will be paid to the details
and to the special needs that will certainly arise? Patients talk to their
students about important concerns that they have. High on the list is
a wish for autonomy, for being in control of decisions about the
course of treatment, the time for stopping therapy and allowing
nature to take its course, and the options open for care when life is
ending. Here, again, students learn that they are to listen to what
patients tell us of themselves and their concepts of self in a world
where control is easily lost.

Parallel to this demand for autonomy, indeed a part of it, is the
expectation for a partnership with the physician, a two-way street of
communication, respect, honesty, and sensitivity that offers the best

that is possible under the conditions of the disease, available therapy, and the possibility of healing. The impressive and important advances in technology can add another barrier to communication by introducing ways of caring for patients that seem to eliminate the person of the caregiver. A strong factor in restoring significant and meaningful communication is the capability of the physician to explain and interpret the disease. In truth, what can the patient know about the options for treatment, the expected outcome, and the impact of the disease and its treatment upon all parts of the life of the patient? What are the anticipated realities of pain and discomfort of treatment, the potential for suffering, economic strain, and a dismal death? What may seem rational to the physician intent upon offering all available treatments even in the face of approaching death can be seen as ludicrous to the patient who understands the inevitable course of the disease leading to that death. These are patient issues and questions that students hear from their teachers as their treatments proceed.

She had had severe diabetes since childhood, along with her parents and siblings. Both parents and one sister had died, and she had only her brother to help her. She had had one leg amputated, and the possibility of a second one was very real. Kidney failure necessitated renal dialysis three times weekly. Fatigue and the dismal prospects for her future convinced her to discontinue dialysis and await her death, cared for by a staff fully understanding of her wishes and her need for companionship on this last journey.

Her medical student was startled by the ease of her decision, impressed with the strength of her resolve.

The most distressing parts of the interactions between student and patient-teacher are the tales of lack of caring, of insensitivity, and of outright disregard for the wishes of patients and their families. Learning the expectations of patients goes a long way in satisfying their hopes for support and understanding at a critical moment in their lives. Insensitivity and lack of awareness, as reported by patients, are strong teaching tools for students as they look forward to their clinical careers. Will they have doubts about their skills, will fatigue or boredom dull their sensibilities, will the burdens of caring for the sick outweigh their hopes for compassion and identification with the hearts and souls of their patients? These questions are not yet answerable, of course, yet sit in their minds as they talk and listen to their patient-teachers.

Seminar Class Experiences

The students meet with me each week in groups of six and discuss their recent interviews. At the beginning of the semester I show several films about the techniques of talking with patients and we discuss their anticipated anxieties about meeting a very sick person. Once the seminar is under way we learn, one by one, the stories of each patient-teacher and the personal responses students make to their conversations, both their feelings and emotions, and the content of the stories. The telling of these highly personal stories gives us insights into how people deal so differently with similar blows to their lives. This is important knowledge for doctors to have: there is no "right" way to understand our final and fateful journey to death. Each of us carries years of experiences, good and bad, positive and negative, fulfilling and degrading, that color our perception of self and others. We can learn of these experiences and of the possible responses persons make to them, and enrich our training so that we can be advocates for our patients whether we agree with their personal philosophies or not.

This learning about the rich variety of the ways we live our lives broadens the student's understanding of what lies ahead in their careers, and offers opportunities for learning to talk with sick persons long before they become responsible for their care. Students comment that they recognize, often for the first time, prejudices and misconceptions in their own minds that could be damaging to their professional lives; their patient-teachers opened their eyes to themselves. They learn to listen and hesitate to be authoritative to someone else, rare behavior among the very bright of this world. The learning about how other persons understand and handle their coming death tells the students of the richness of human diversity, and the need for physicians to honor these differences for the better care of the patient and the enrichment of the person of the doctor.

In listening to classmates discuss their experiences with their patients we all learn the delicate skills that are so essential to learning about the lives of others. We bring our own inherent differences to these meetings, and we can hear new ways to listen, new approaches to sensitive and personal issues, the values of paying close attention to what is said. An interesting side benefit is hearing how patients interpret what the doctor and nurse have said or not said; patients hang on every word they hear, dissecting with great care all the possible ramifications of each word. Again, for the student this is invaluable information. We must be explicit, clear, and careful in what we say to patients, speaking with kindness and support to concerns that are absolutely essential to the patient.

The medical student was sitting in the examining room talking with the young man with leukemia. His college career had been abruptly halted by this disease and its protracted treatments, but he was hopeful that he would return to school soon. As they talked, a resident physician came and stood in the doorway, facing halfway into the room. He said "hello," reported the latest blood count, and, with some hesitation, outlined the pills the patient was to take, and when. He said that the young man was free to call him if he had questions. After he left, the patient was silent. The attending physician then came into the room, sat down next to the young man, and put his hand on his shoulder. He, in almost identical words, reported the blood count, and went over the treatment schedule with great care, writing down the names of the drugs and the times they were to be taken. He wrote down his telephone number, told him to call anytime, and asked if he had any questions. He said "goodbye and good luck," and left with a handshake.

The young man turned to the student and said that the resident was the worst, and the attending the best doctor he knew. Although both had said essentially the same words, their personal demeanor defined their place in this young man's mind. The student understood the differences and took them to her heart.

Defining the Ideals

Students comment that the seminar gives them an opportunity to define and discuss the reasons why they are in medical school. Their experiences with their patient-teachers clarify for them what are often vague ideas about doing good, caring for others, and relieving suffering. Now, as new students with no medical knowledge or experience, they are learning what it means to be a person, often like a parent or a grandparent, who is very sick. This entails a confrontation with the self, with concepts of personhood, responsibility, duties, and compassion. For many of us, this is a central track in learning to be a good doctor. The grasp we get that we are a human being caring for other human beings, not a doctor treating a patient can be, in these early years of training, an instruction not to be forgotten. The patient-teachers offer perspectives on the profession of medicine that is not available elsewhere, giving the students the chance to redefine, restate, and confirm their commitments to a profession that is always in need of review and revision. The medical student continued his reflections on his time spent with his patient-teacher, Rose.

I just couldn't seem to salvage Rose as I waited for the elevator and all I could think was that she should go home and die. Not here in this dreary hospital with dimmed lights. But as the elevator let me out and I walked among the action through the lovely fountained atrium a new phrase came to my mind and repeated like a mantra— *red rose, proud rose, sad rose of all my days.* That's a Yeats line and it caught something inside me that was falling.

From the day we are born until we die/Is but the winking of an eye. That's another Yeats line. I know Yeats was melodramatic, but I love him. With him, the seeds of doom and tragedy grow to passion. *I cast my heart into my rhymes,* he continues, *that you in the dim coming times/May know how my heart went with them/After the red rose bordered hem.* . . . But if we cast, oh if we cast, Rose, we can defy our boundaries. Defiance, that's the net that's catching me. I cast, I cast my heart. Sad Rose, red Rose, but also proud, proud Rose. Pushing the pain meds button without the hope of a drop. A gesture with which to brighten these dim hospital lights. Push the button, Rose, cast your thumb down upon that old Atari joystick and catch the world, the dim coming times. Such a fish as will break the hearts of many. The broken heart of passion and rage, cast redly, proudly, sadly, for all our days.[4]

Notes

1. E. Choo, personal communication, 1996.
2. F. Balamuth, personal communication, 1996.
3. D. Jacoby, personal communication, 1996.
4. Ibid.

10

The Realized Life of the Physician

Who shall say what prospect life offers to another? Could a greater miracle take place than for us to look through each other's eyes for an instant? We should live in all the ages of the world in an hour; ay, in all the worlds of the ages. History, Poetry, Mythology!—I know of no reading of another's experience so startling and informing as this would be.

Henry David Thoreau, *Walden*[1]

An ideal found in much of literature over the many centuries of our common history is the hope for a good life, a life that offers a conviction of fulfillment in work done, relationships known and cherished, pleasures and joys experienced, and that certainty that the life lived was a valid one. For many of us over these millennia, perhaps for most, these have been empty dreams ending all too soon in early death from disease and violence, stunted lives lived in poverty and starvation, in slavery in its many forms, and hope destroyed by prejudice and hate. There are a few professions, however, that have offered, from time immemorial, the possibilities of a realized life; a dedicated profession that grants opportunities for valid work, affec-

145

tion and respect, and gratitude for the gifts of caring for others. Over these many years of our history the priest and the physician—by whatever names they are known in our widely differing cultures—have been given the possibility of a realized life. Obviously, there have been countless persons outside these professions who have led an exemplary life graced with all the gifts one could desire, and many within these professions have been miserable and evil members of their society. But healers and spiritual guides have been given opportunities for the good life beyond ordinary expectations.

Shamans and healers, and we who share these callings in our own cultures, have the profound privilege of being with and for others in their times of suffering, despair, self-denigration, and sadness. We also are with those nearly overwhelmed with thankfulness and joy, freedom, and the gift of a second chance that begins a new lease on life. There is such a potential for enrichment and fulfillment of the self of the physician and the pastor in the work and companionship offered by their professions. Medicine, in particular, plays a special role in human culture, especially in Western culture. There are opportunities in medicine for realizing three outstanding hopes of young persons today: work that serves important, and often critical, needs of others; ongoing contact with the fascinating and rapidly developing physical sciences; and the financial and social rewards that assure a good lifestyle. Certainly the large number of applicants to medical schools attests to the popularity of the profession even in times of uncertainty about the ways in which medical care will be provided in the immediate future, the methods and the amounts of remuneration for services, and the potentialities for research in the medical sciences. Despite these questions, the practice of medicine remains a highly desirable and idealistic goal for many. It is so, I believe, because it offers those rare opportunities in our world to be with and for other persons in times of distress, anxiety, and the unwelcome exigencies of sickness, genetic misfortune, accident, and the inevitability of death.

It is sometimes forgotten how remarkably doctors enter the lives of their patients. The routine personal history inquires into aspects of another individual that are absolutely out of bounds for any other person to ask. We assume that both pastor and doctor will assure the patient or parishioner that any truthful statement or confession is held in confidence except in those most urgent of situations where the life of another is threatened. The physical examination takes for granted the touching of the body of another in places and ways unimaginable except in the most intimate relationship. Yet we think nothing of it, either as patient or physician, knowing that accuracy of diagnosis is dependent upon as complete a revelation of the whole person as is possible, by physical examination as well as by history, including psychological, cultural, sexual, and social aspects of being a person. In the daily practice of medicine these conditions are accepted as integral to accurate care, and in many instances there is certainly no pressing requirement for a complete evaluation of the psychological, social, or religious status of patients. But, knowing as we do that doctor and patient can have distinctly different agendas about the nature of the consultation, it is important that all caregivers be alert to signals that there are other issues than the presenting complaint. When serious disease or accident raises questions about survival or the need for difficult, prolonged, and painful treatments whose outcomes are questionable, attention must be paid to personal issues as well as the medical ones. When death is a considered possibility, problems arise for many doctors, complicating relationships with the patient and the family.

Problems Posed by Dying Persons

In a 1988 "Sounding Board" article in the *New England Journal of Medicine* Egilde P. Seravalli writes,

> Every physician has a professional mandate to help other human beings in need. But the inevitability of a patient's death may challenge this code, unless the physician is willing to add a new dimension to the patient-doctor relationship: that of helping the patient deal with the experience of dying. . . . The presence of the doctor in this last phase of life may be crucial for a peaceful death. It can allow the patient not only to die with self-respect, but also to feel less lonely.[2]

As has been noted before, doctors can have mixed emotions around the care of the dying, raising, as it does, those exquisitely sensitive concerns for their own mortality. There is a universal fear of death brought to consciousness by attending the dying. The death of another person, particularly a patient one has known for a long time, provides an unwelcome view of our own future, confirming the one-way road we are on from birth to death. While this is true for all persons, it seems to have a weightier impact upon the physician, a reminder of the final failure of medicine to heal. As physicians this sense of failure can be internalized. Jonathan Lieff, M.D., a psychiatrist at Boston University School of Medicine, writes,

> When dealing with a difficult elderly and dying patient, the doctor may experience a psychological impotence. Doctors are not taught a clear method for helping patients accept death. Rather, doctors are taught to keep people alive at all costs and strive to work with patients in an optimistic and confident manner, in order to instill confidence in patients. The feeling of helplessness in the face of death is difficult for a doctor to handle, thereby making it easier to turn away from such patients than to accept defeat.[3]

Most of us are ill at ease in a variety of circumstances: meeting someone with whom we have had an argument; speaking with a friend or spouse about unacceptable behavior; confronting another person about an obligation; and bearing bad news. This latter task is one of the functions of the doctor, and one that has been discussed, mostly from the side of the bearer, not the receiver, of the bad news. There are almost no empirical studies of the ways in which bad news is given, and most of the articles about this issue are by physicians, not patients. Some suggestions about breaking bad news are offered in a review of the literature by J. T. Placek and Tara L. Eberhardt in *JAMA*, the *Journal of the American Medical Association,* in 1996. They point out obvious conditions that should be met: the location of the meeting, the necessity of it being done in person and in the presence of supportive family or friends, the allowance of enough time for explanation and discussion, a translation of scientific terms into understandable language, and the inclusion of some suggestions of hope. In their analysis they comment on the two perceptions we have when given bad news: an appraisal of the situation by what is known about the disease, and a second appraisal of the resources available to cope. "Events that are appraised as threatening and as severely depleting or exceeding one's resources are most likely to be perceived as stressful. Perceptions of stress are then met with some conscious attempt to cope."[4] Obviously the physician plays the major role in making these appraisals as positive and as helpful as possible.

An important factor in telling bad news, and one that impedes the process, is a sense of discomfort physicians know when they feel powerless to cure, when they are talking with a person who will die of this disease. One of the causes of this discomfort can be not knowing what the patient considers the significance of the diagnosis and the prognosis. Most studies of telling bad news are one-sided in that they are reports of the experiences of the doctors, not the patients. An important qualifier in this process is taking the time to learn from the patient the meanings of the diagnosis, and not infer those meanings from a projection of what the diagnosis might mean to the doctor. Age, experience, relationships, profession, religious conviction, and knowledge will profoundly determine what the diagnosis means. Certainly, the diagnosis of acute leukemia will have a different impact upon a twenty-five-year-old single parent of two children than it will upon a seventy-five-year-old retired doctor and grandfather. Knowing the patient, learning the details of past encounters with critical issues, and asking the right questions can make a difference to the patient. This method can also grace the doctor with some assurance that the covenant between them will be fulfilled by the mutual understandings they share of the work to be done.

The Work of the Physician

"Sickness" and "healing" are two words central to the ways in which physicians and surgeons understand the work of caring for patients. In the Introduction to his book, *Sickness and Healing*, Robert A. Hahn offers workable definitions of these words. He writes,

[T]he essence of "sickness" is an unwanted condition in one's person or self—one's mind, body, soul, or connection to the world. What counts as "sickness" is thus determined by the perception and experience of its bearer, the patient (from the Latin *pati-*, as in "passion," to suffer, to bear affliction). Sicknesses represent and express the particularities of individual patients within a society.[5]

The cultural environment of the patient is of extreme importance to the physician since our understanding of all that matters to us is so determined by our cultural heritage through family, religion, language, and experience. The impact of sickness upon us is radically defined by this inheritance, and must be a strong factor in interpretation of a diagnosis and the prospects for treatments and recovery. As we know, an annoyance to one can be a near-catastrophe to another. The significance of an upper respiratory infection for an opera singer is considerably different from that for a computer operator. In like manner, we can understand disease as divine punishment, as pure chance, as a result of ignorance and improper diet and habits, and as the inevitable winnowing that includes us all when life is to end.

For the physician, healing is the primary goal of medical care, although prevention of disease is probably the more effective way to ensure health and longevity in our world. Again, Hahn defines healing as "the redress of sickness." He continues, "I include as healing not only the remedy or cure for sickness—that is, the restoration of a prior healthy state—but also rehabilitation—the compensation for loss of health—and palliation—the mitigation of suffering in the sick."[6] He goes on to point out that not all who regard themselves as healers do heal. We know well the prevalence of iatrogenic disorders, self-serving operative procedures, and errors in diagnosis and treatment that occur. It is recognized in many cultures that other factors—environmental, social, spiritual, and psychological—can heal when traditional medicine cannot. Even a superficial knowledge of anthropology qualifies any simple conviction that Western medicine is the answer to the problems of health in our world. The profound differences among peoples in their definitions of sickness, notions of healing, understanding of death, and expectations for life should make us wary of assuming that Western medicine is the answer. Rather, we are to learn from our patients what is expected of us as purported healers, and what patients understand to be their role in their own care.

Understanding the social connections of patients can be a major factor in their care as well as their cure. This aspect of medicine is not well understood by many doctors, but is important for many in determining sickness and health. Hahn, commenting on a ten-year study in Alameda County, California, from 1965 to 1975, writes,

> Even when factors such as health status in 1965, risk behavior . . . , socioeconomic status, and preventive healthcare practices were taken into account, persons least connected with others were still more than twice as likely to have died in the ten-year interval than persons who were more connected with others. The persistence of an association between social connectedness and mortality . . . suggests both that social connectedness is a precursor rather than (or in addition to) a result of poor health and that the effect of connectedness is independent of other major risk factors for death.[7]

We know that recent widows and widowers have a much higher risk of death in their time of mourning than they would have were the spouse still alive. These findings are important to health care and need to be part of the general knowledge of all caregivers in treatment, in preventive medicine, and in planning both future care and education of students.

It might be instructive to look at the patient-doctor covenant or relationship in a reversal of the popular model of the doctor being the more important partner, possessing knowledge and experience accrued over years of education and training. It could be an advantage to all if the patient were understood as the driving force in the relationship, with demands and expectations for care, for caring, for playing a significant role in planning and managing that care. This would entail, of course, the expectation that the patient would accept that role. Many persons are happy to turn their care over to others, abdicating their rights and their responsibilities to care for themselves. One of the roles that the doctor can step into is to encourage the patient to assume those duties as far as it is possible to do so.

An inhibitor to cementing the bond between patient and doctor, as noted previously, is the environment within which the students learn by observing the behavior of attending physicians and house staff. George Annas, commenting about the SUPPORT study published in *JAMA* in 1995, writes that doctors do not take the rights of hospitalized patients seriously.

> The most central reason is that in the modern teaching hospital, patient care is often a distant third goal after teaching and research. In the high-tech, high pressure environment, there is little room for thoughtfulness, for the intrusion of human values, or for conversation with the patient or family. . . . Medical students and residents are taught that talking is a waste of time, distracting them from the time available to do real medicine. And when even doing real medicine cannot help the dying patient, students and residents quickly learn that the attendings are uninterested in having discussions with patients or families about death or pain.[8]

In these times of change in the management of health care, the pressures of economic forces and greed on that care, and scientific advances that offer amazing new possibilities for diagnosis and treatment, the simple duties of "attending" to patients are easily lost. This possibility makes all the more critical the need for the physician to evaluate—indeed, to revalue—the goals of the personal and the professional lives being lived. An example of this need to continually assess the means of proper and sensitive care for patients is the 1997 report of a study at Johns Hopkins on the effects of bedside case presentations on how patients perceive their care. Compared to conference room presentations, well-educated patients noted that the staff spent more time with them and explained their diseases and treatments more fully at the bedside. There is a serious caveat in the report: less well-educated patients found complex medical terminology a stumbling block, pointing strongly to the need to improve communication. The report concludes, "Bedside presentations . . . provide a unique opportunity for students to learn from both patients and experienced clinicians. According to many, bedside is the ideal place to teach the art and science of medical examination."[9]

The Search for the Realized Life

Physicians and surgeons—those for whom the care of patients is a significant part of their professional life—have the real potential for living a life, the quality of which is possible for very few other persons. They are in an intellectual community for which science provides a rational base for understanding their work and increasing their knowledge and understanding; they are in constant contact with other human beings in varied states of need, usually considered important, often serious, and occasionally life-threatening. Why, then, are many doctors dissatisfied with their work, distanced from, even angry at, their patients, and subject to growing distrust by the public? Granted, recent changes in the economics of health care and increasing management of the profession by persons outside of it committed to goals not necessarily related to patient care have caused major strains. But medicine remains a very attractive career for undergraduate students, and medicine retains its high status as a moral profession dedicated to service. As noted before, it is not that everyone else is pleased with their particular profession and work, basking in honors bestowed by the public. But many doctors, given the admirable characteristics of the profession, are unhappy with it.

I would suggest that a major source of these difficulties lies in the failure of the training of doctors in appropriate care of the seriously ill patient. By appropriate care I mean comprehensive engagement of the physician in the personal concerns, attitudes, and convictions of persons in their care. This is not a simplistic suggestion. I am well aware of the difficulties in involving oneself in the lives of others. There are many impressive challenges to this work, and a number of potential pitfalls are evident. But these are resolvable with studied thought and willingness to extend the self to others in ways other than, yet obviously including, providing a diagnosis and prescribed treatments. The returns on the investments in time and energy are considerable, and offer to fulfill the hopes we all have for living a significant and rewarding life. There needs to be education of students and staff in the ways and means of communication with patients and with colleagues in the healthcare profession that recognize the deep needs we all have for community, for care that is sensitive to us as unique persons, and companionship on that last journey we will all take to our death.

The sad aspect to this problem of the difficulty in learning how to be engaged in the personal components of patient care is the loss that caregivers suffer when they cannot meet the obvious needs that patients voice for signs of compassion and sympathy. Not only do patients fail to receive assurances of comfort and companionship when they are sick and dying; doctors also lose a significant gift of enrichment and contentment at having stayed with another person during the awesome and difficult time before death. If there is any parallel human experience that can instruct us about learning to be with and for the dying, I think that it is learning to love. The word *love* has many meanings: the ultimate expression of being the giving of one's life for a friend. I use it here to describe the affection, cooperation, and sacrifice we associate with a fulfilling and rewarding family relationship of generations of persons responding with affection and care for each other, or other similar long-term relationships and friendships that express commitment and willingness to give as well as receive. The Greek word *agape* seems to capture the essence of this type of love in Christian history. Common experience confirms that, if we are to be graced with these gifts of love, we must give of ourselves. In fact, the more that we give of ourselves, the more we seem to get. There is a relationship established in which the bread cast upon the waters returns to us increased.

I venture the observation that the depth of our relationships with seriously ill and dying patients will reflect back to us in deepened self-knowledge, strengthened abilities to work even more sensitively with future patients, and a profound satisfaction at having been a physician all the way with one who asked for our presence. If we, as caregivers, could make the effort that Thoreau suggests we do—"look through each other's eyes for an instant"—we might well learn the depths of meaning we could incorporate for ourselves. We also could, at least partially, try to grasp the significance of the illnesses we witness daily on our rounds. Willingness to stay with the very sick is a clear marker for the developing and realized self, a person secure enough in professional skill and interior integrity to stay with patients through their ordeals and their release. These are what I define as spiritual acts: the recognition and acceptance of a part of the human personality beyond body and mind that upholds us in our weakness and failure, that unites us with that recognizable spark of life in all others, and which, finally, transcends the world we know. Patricia A. Marshall, associate director of the medical humanities program at Loyola University, writes in the *Hastings Center Report*,

> The relationship between dying patients and their physicians can be the source of a profound recognition of the strength and durability of the human spirit. A healing relationship transcends the gravity and finality of pain and suffering because it implies something more than a technical consideration of the physical and mortal body.[10]

There is a long history in the religions of this world that speaks to the commonality of human life from its birth to its death. We bring nothing into the world and we shall certainly take nothing out of it. But, if we can live that life in compassionate service using our skills to the best of our abilities, we will have accomplished more than most have in our history.

The Patient as Our Teacher

It is amazing that, as recently as 1997, medical journals carry articles expressing the hope that doctors will learn to be able to talk with their patients in ways that recognize the emotional content of speech. A piece in *JAMA* in February 1997 describes a method for interpreting conversational lapses and missing signals. The conclusion of the paper is that

> the basic empathic skills seem to be recognizing when emotions may be present but not directly expressed, inviting exploration of these unexpressed feelings, and effectively acknowledging these feelings so the patient feels understood. The frequent lack of acknowledgment by physicians of both direct and indirect expressions of affect poses a threat to the patient-physician relationship. . . .[11]

From my experiences over the past twelve years with the Seminar on the Seriously Ill Patient, I know these skills can be learned from the patient. The persistent problem is the inability or the unwillingness of the physician to listen to the story the patient has to tell. There are, in these stories, innumerable hints, innuendos, casual references, and outright statements that beg for questioning and exploration. And it is the patient, via the narrative of self-revelation, and not another doctor, who can teach us what we need to know about caring for the very sick and comforting the dying.

We all have a history, a one-of-a-kind account of our lives that has been influenced by a wide variety of factors, most of which will play a part in how we respond to all the events that we will encounter. As noted before, culture, religion, family structure, ethnicity and race, states of mental and physical health, occupation, education, and countless other aspects of being a person determine how we will understand and function. All of these varied characteristics can be learned from patients as we care for them. Not only is the individual person benefited by our interest and concern; we learn from patients how to do the questioning and interpret the answers to the benefit of that patient and others who will follow. One of the key learning experiences for the caregiver is the futility of making judgments on the values, lifestyles, and beliefs of others. Not that we would accept them as our own ways of living; but the concern of the physician is the care of the patient, a developed understanding of this individual at this moment in time in need of attention. If changes in lifestyle will improve the health and welfare of the patient, suggestions and instructions for change should be offered as part of therapy, including finding the supports needed to implement change.

One of the lessons students learn in the seminar is the great variation in personality found in their patients. It is obvious that there is not a single way to deal with the problems of sickness, loss, and death. There are many different approaches that we take as we adjust to bad news and frightening probabilities, and these can be learned from our patients who teach us this variety. The patients also teach us the depth of the human spirit, the function of faith in confronting the many problems of disease and disability, and the resilience that we can muster to see us through bad times. It is this process of learning that enriches the caregiver by teaching what others know and do so that we can help others with a range of possibilities and not a stunted, single-minded view of reality.

In their experience in this seminar, which occurs at the beginning of their medical education, students learn that conversation with sick persons is usually easy, is appreciated by patients, and grants the student an inside track in that person's life. Patients are very open with students, knowing that they are intent upon learning how to speak with patients about the central concerns of their illness, however intimate and personal they might be. A third-year student who had taken the seminar his first year was doing his surgical rotation. He was the type of person who would note the photographs on the bedside table, the cards drawn by a grandchild on the wall, introduce himself to visitors and family. On rounds that morning with the attending surgeon, a visiting professor, the house staff, charge nurse, social worker, and other students, the surgeon told the patient assigned to this student of the plan to do a certain procedure as part of treatment. The patient listened intently, asked a question or two, and then said that she would have to ask her doctor about this. The startled attending surgeon said, "But *I* am your doctor!" The patient turned and pointed to the student: "He is my doctor."

Comment

Henry David Thoreau calls his readers to awaken, to discover their lives in this world.

> Morning is when I am awake and there is dawn in me. . . . We must learn to reawaken and keep ourselves awake, not by mechanical aids, but by an infinite expectation of the dawn, which does not forsake us in our soundest sleep. I know of no more encouraging fact than the unquestionable ability of man to elevate his life by a conscious endeavor.[12]

We are called to awaken to the possibilities we have for a developed and a realized life. For those of us who care for others in their sicknesses and personal crises and accidents, we have an opportunity rarely offered others to enrich our lives while offering comfort and companionship to others. The ones who teach us to care and to mature in mind and spirit are our patients, those farther along on the road of life. Their experiences and thoughts, their emotions and relationships, their limitations and insights, their suffering and pain, their acceptance and understanding are gifts to us that are priceless for our own growth. They teach us that we may also give of ourselves, becoming the richer for it.

Notes

1. Henry David Thoreau, *Walden,* ed. by J. Lyndon Shanley (Princeton, N.J.: Princeton University Press, 1971), 10.

2. Egilde Seravalli, "The Dying Patient, the Physician, and the Fear of Death," *New England Journal of Medicine* 319, no. 26 (December 1988): 1729.

3. Jonathan Lieff, "Eight Reasons Why Doctors Fear the Elderly, Chronic Illness, and Death," *Journal of Transpersonal Psychology* 14, no. 1 (1982): 58.

4. J. T. Placek and Tara L. Eberhardt, "Breaking Bad News," *JAMA* 276, no. 6 (August 14, 1996): 499.

5. Robert A. Hahn, *Sickness and Healing* (New Haven: Yale University Press, 1995), 5.

6. Ibid., 7.

7. Ibid., 87.

8. George J. Annas, "How We Lie," Special Supplement, *Hastings Center Report* 25, no. 6 (1995): S12.

9. L. S. Lehmann, F. L. Brancati, M-C. Chen, D. Roter, and A. S. Dobs, "The Effect of Bedside Case Presentations on Patient's Perceptions of Their Medical Care," *NEJM,* 336, no. 16 (April 17, 1997): 1155.

10. Patricia A. Marshall, "The SUPPORT Study: Who's Talking?" Special Supplement, *Hastings Center Report* 25, no. 6 (1995): S11.

11. Anthony L. Suchman, Kathryn Markakis, Howard B. Beckman, and Richard Frankel, "A Model of Empathic Communication in the Medical Interview," *JAMA* 277, no. 8 (February 26, 1997): 678.

12. Thoreau, *Walden,* 90.

11

Postscript

These are times of change in medical care. Two of the major factors are the shift of the provision of care to corporate organizations—managed care in its varied forms—and rapid developments in technology that offer new and impressive methods of diagnosis, treatment, and sustenance of the physiological functions of the human body. These developments cause changes in both the professions that care for sick persons and in the patient population seeking care. There are many nearly visible and probable procedures and therapies that will have profound implications both for the professions and for their patients. Gene therapy and other probable techniques being explored in the field of genetics are on the horizon. Amazing new procedures for producing images of the interior of the body, for performing surgery with minimal injury, and for operating on fetuses for repair of congenital defects are occurring almost daily.

From the perspective of the patient, there is a modicum of disquiet and discontent with traditional medicine. An impressive increase in the number of persons choosing alternative-treatment options from a variety of healers is quite obvious. Communication between doctor and patient, never considered to be generally excellent, is an ongoing focus of irritation for persons seeking care. The old days of paternalism, of "doctor knows best," are gone, and patients are more demanding in learning about their medical problems and in questioning what the profession is considering for action.

A prominent contemporary concern in the United States is care of the patient when life is coming to a close. The care of the seriously ill and the dying person is now a topic of general conversation, increasingly so as the role of the physician in assisting persons to die is debated by the profession, by the courts, and by the public. The moral, ethical, and practical concerns are nearly overwhelming, involving, as they do, religious, societal, cultural, and psychological centers of our lives by which we live and make our decisions about who we are with each other.

It would be nice if there were some simple and workable solutions to these questions, but they are not readily visible. In the meantime, there are patients to be cared for by doctors, physician associates, nurses, social workers, and a broad range of technicians. How do we learn to care for very sick persons so that both their medical and personal needs and the personal and professional goals and expectations of their caregivers will be met? What, if any, are the skills and the techniques for accomplishing both goals—patient care and professional satisfaction? Aside from the critical education that must be mastered by students before they begin their professional work, how can students on their ways to becoming practitioners learn to become the compassionate and loyal caregivers they aspire to be in their fruitful futures?

In this study I have considered at some length the many problems we face when we are very sick. Suffering, in its multiple modes and guises, is a common part of the experiences we know with disease. We suffer in body, mind, and spirit, and these are fateful areas for concern by family and friends, as well as by the professions caring for the sick. The provision of good care will require a certain identification with the sick person, seeing in that person the plight of all of us, a forthright example of the road we will all travel in the future. The patient is central in this study and should be our primary concern, indeed our teacher.

Those who provide care are important also because their talents, their empathy, their self-understanding will determine their capacities for caring appropriately in the times of difficulty and stress; and, caring with the rewards of satisfaction with work well done and with the gifts of awareness of self-fulfillment and gratitude from patients. In my experiences over the past sixteen years as chaplain to the Yale University School of Medicine, I have learned from students and from faculty about these complex, yet straightforward concerns. In response to a recognized and voiced need of students to learn how to become good doctors in the personal and emotional senses, I developed a course, the Seminar on the Seriously Ill Patient, for helping students learn the issues and the concerns of very sick patients. After three decades of my own medical practice as a pediatrician, this course and my interactions with students, their patient-teachers, nurses, and faculty have been of profound importance for my own proceeding development as a person.

The focus of the course is the use of sick patients as teachers, one-on-one, with first-year medical students. The patients help the students learn about the interior, personal aspects of disease, and the impact of that disease upon a life in all its varied parts. The hope is that this will be the beginning of a long and fruitful journey of education and self-knowledge that will provide the basis for a fully realized life as a doctor. But it is not only the student who learns in this course. Patients also comment on the self-understanding they have experienced as they describe their lives: their medical, surgical, and treatment experiences; their responses to them; their supports (or lack of same); their awareness of both the character and the characteristics of the good physician.

I have described the course in some detail, including comments by students and my observations on their growth and development during the course. And these observations and hopes that I have for the students are forerunners for the distant goal of helping the physicians of tomorrow work toward a life that is enriched and worthy, adjusting to the ever-changing and varied challenges presented both by patients and by the society and the culture in which they live and, often, suffer. To become a good doctor aware of the needs of others, prepared to listen and respond as a compassionate person to another who is ill, and to find satisfaction and realization in this work—that is the purpose of this study.

Henry David Thoreau, with his sharp concern for awakening to the dawn that is ever present for us, has been a constant companion of mine during my years of practice, study, and chaplaincy. His persistent demand—or plea—that we become what we can become, that we learn who we are and where we are going have been guidelines for me. We must persist in being alert to our world of nature *and* in in-depth study of the self. These goals seem to me to be essential for becoming a good doctor.